# The Spirited Walker

# The
# *Spirited Walker*

FITNESS WALKING

for

CLARITY,

BALANCE,

and

SPIRITUAL CONNECTION

## CAROLYN SCOTT KORTGE

HarperSanFrancisco

*A Division of* HarperCollins*Publishers*

Grateful acknowledgment is made to the following for permission to reprint material copyrighted or controlled by them:

Lines from "The Way In" ("Eingang") by Rainer Maria Rilke from the book *Selected Poems of Rainer Maria Rilke,* translated by Robert Bly, copyright © 1981 by Robert Bly. Reprinted by permission of HarperCollins Publishers, Inc.

"The Task" by Eugene Guillevic from *Selected Poems.* Copyright © 1969 by Denise Levertov Goodman and Eugene Guillevic. Reprinted by permission of New Directions Publishing Corp.

Lines from "The Path is You," from the book *The Long Road Turns to Joy: A Guide to Walking Meditation,* by Thich Nhat Hanh, copyright © 1996 by Thich Nhat Hanh. Reprinted by permission of Parallax Press.

Excerpt from "The Invocation to Kali, Part 5," copyright © 1971 by May Sarton from the book *Collected Poems 1930–1993,* by May Sarton. Reprinted by permission of W. W. Norton & Company, Inc.

"The Last Shall be First," by George Sheehan, from *Runner's World* magazine, Vol. 27, No. 8, August 1992, and from the book *Going the Distance* by George Sheehan, copyright © 1996 by The George Sheehan Trust. Reprinted by permission of George Sheehan III and The George Sheehan Trust.

---

Illustrations by Kenge Kobayashi

HarperCollins Web Site: http://www.harpercollins.com

HarperCollins®, 🐚 ®, and HarperSanFrancisco™ are trademarks of HarperCollins Publishers, Inc.

HarperCollins books may be purchased for educational, business, or sales promotional use. For information please write: Special Markets Department, HarperCollins Publishers, Inc., 10 East 53rd Street, New York, NY 10022.

FIRST EDITION

Library of Congress Cataloging-in-Publication Data

Kortge, Carolyn Scott.
    The spirited walker : fitness walking for clarity, balance, and spiritual connection / Carolyn Scott Kortge. — 1st ed.
        p.   cm.
    Includes bibliographical references and index.
    ISBN 0–06–064736–1 (pbk.)
    1. Fitness walking.  2. Fitness walking—psychological aspects.
I. Title.
RA781.65.K67   1998
613.7'176—dc21                                                                 97-49217

98 99 00 01 02 ❖/RRD 10 9 8 7 6 5 4 3 2 1

*To Dean,*
*My favorite walking companion*

# CONTENTS

# Contents

# INTRODUCTION

## *Border Crossings*

For most of my life, a picture of awkwardness dominated my mind whenever I approached a physical challenge. In it, I gripped the handlebars of my first bicycle in frozen terror as I teetered down a gravel alley. The memory kept me off balance and made me wary of physical risks. As an adult, I hid my discomfort behind disclaimers and self-deprecating humor. "I've never been athletic," I'd shrug as I grappled with golf clubs and ski poles. Clumsiness seemed my destiny, as natural and non-negotiable as the genetic code that produced my brown hair.

In the 1970s, I sampled jogging. "It'll get better after the first mile," enthusiastic friends promised. It didn't and I quit. I took aerobics classes like vitamin pills—because they were good for me. Then, in the 1980s, I caught the curl of the fitness-walking wave and discovered for the first time in my life an athletic pursuit that I was good at. I became a dedicated fitness walker and set off on a journey that has brought me much more than the physical workout I'd hoped for.

The journey began with a departure so simple and undramatic that it gave no clue to the adventures ahead. My job as a newspaper feature writer required a sharp eye for trends. When walking appeared on the fitness horizon as an alternative to running and aerobics classes, I covered the story. I wrote about the formation of walking clubs and detailed the merits of low-impact workouts. Soon I'd measured a two-mile route in my neighborhood and embarked on my own experiments with this "new" fitness option. Before long, I had made a commitment to meet friends before work on Friday mornings for a walk in a hilly section of town. Even at a pedestrian pace, we'd work up a sweat before breakfast. In no time, I was badgering them to walk with me in a three-mile community run on Saint Patrick's Day.

The ease and enthusiasm with which I found my own stride in the emerging walking movement surprised me. It almost seemed out of character for a woman who had stubbornly maintained a nonathletic status for forty years. When I was growing up, girls learned early in life to guard against physical exertion. In PE classes, no one spurred us to explore the range of our physical strength and potential. No one encouraged us to sweat. Most of us stumbled through volleyball and calisthenics, convinced we weren't meant to be athletic.

But walking crept under my defenses. Walking seemed so simple. I had no idea that these external steps would launch an internal expedition. Step by step, walking drew me into an adventure that traveled unmapped corners myself. Internal boundaries shifted. The tight lines that had bound me inside the image of an athletic "klutz" began to loosen. Instead of a klutz, I found a woman who loved testing her physical limits. She liked feeling active and strong. I hadn't known that about myself. For years, I had been looking at my body from the outside, as something to control with discipline and diet. When I stepped inside, I connected with a new self-image and a deeper knowledge of myself.

"We are each, inside us, a country with our own mountains and plateaus and chasms and storms and seas of tranquility, but like a Third World country we remain largely unexplored, and sometimes even impoverished, for want of a little investment," writer Dorothy Gilman observed.[1] Walking introduced unexpected opportunities for me to make an investment in myself. It offered an exploration of internal mountains, plateaus, chasms, and storms that I'd never glimpsed. It changed my perspective and revealed a wholeness I hadn't known before. A part of me that delights in movement had been hidden from my view.

For a time, the discovery carried me into an exhilarating world of stopwatches and athletic training. At an age when most athletes have retired, I entered my first track meet. *I am here and I am strong,* I chanted in rhythm with my feet when self-doubt slowed my pace. *I am here and I can do this.* Steps and words forged an alliance. They emerged in an integration of muscles, mind, and spirit that restored connection between parts of myself that had been at odds for many years.

Then the journey brought me home again, a fitness walker traveling the sidewalks of my neighborhood. But like a tourist whose life has been changed by the sights and impressions encountered on an unforgettable adventure, I came home a different person. *I am here and I am strong,* I told myself as I moved through walking workouts. *I am here and I am clear. Clear and strong and calm.* Words and phrases that affirmed my strength as a walker also had significance for me as a woman, a writer, a friend. My steps had led to a spiritual path that travels from sole to soul.

The route that leads through body to spirit is already familiar to many athletes. Twenty-five years ago Esalen Institute cofounder Michael Murphy identified a "spiritual underground" in sports. His interviews with top athletes revealed a side of physical performance seldom covered on the sports pages.[2] But even if I had read his work then, I wouldn't have understood it. And I most certainly wouldn't have imagined that an ordinary fitness walker could aspire to the same experience. I would have been wrong. Access to the "spiritual underground" of sports isn't achieved by setting world records or winning gold medals. It is reached with practice.

Practice lets you begin wherever you are and move forward at your own pace, knowing that progress builds steadily. Meditators recognize that a regular practice of mindfulness increases their ability to clear the mind of self-talk and distraction. Musicians depend on consistent practice to reach the heights of harmony. Athletes master physical excellence with frequent training sessions. Practice makes patterns; it etches habits into our cells. All practice is mental as well as physical. And the reverse is also true; movement in the body brings movement in the mind. It is a natural alchemy.

So many of us seek this kind of movement in our lives, a fusion of being and doing. We long to restore wholeness within ourselves and to connect with one another and with the spiritual values that sustain and guide us. A few years ago I would have thought it absurd if someone had told me that walking could transform a life in this way. You may have similar doubts. I hope you'll find inspiration here, along with practical techniques for starting or enriching your own walking program.

Experiment with new ways of walking and new ways of thinking. Draw inspiration from my experiences and from the stories of other walkers who appear throughout the book. Their steps have carried them across continents and through personal tragedies. They've walked for causes and for recovery. They've toured the canyons inside themselves, finding direction from the sole up.

Regardless of your starting speed or fitness level, the route to inner and outer movement can begin on a walking path. Whatever your motivation for walking—relaxation, aerobic fitness, weight loss, a healthy heart, or interaction with nature—a spirited walk can become the first step of a spiritual journey.

# CHAPTER 1

## *In Step*

### Fitness for Body, Mind, and Spirit

It had turned into one of those too-familiar days. Demands and disruptions had left the schedule in shambles. By the time I tied my walking shoes, the early dusk of a winter afternoon hovered on the horizon. It would be dark before I rounded the corner at the midway mark of my usual neighborhood loop. As soon as I hit the street, my mind started planning dinner and scanning cupboards, pushing to squeeze fitness and food into a tight time slot. *I am here and I am walking,* I reminded myself mentally, pulling my attention to the present and to a fast, rhythmic walking pace. *I am here and I am breathing.*

Twenty minutes out, I rounded the corner and turned toward home. Now the wind that had followed my steps met me head on, slapping at my face and taunting me with a splattering of rain. *No,* my brain screamed. *No! Not now! No rain! No wind! I'm tired. I shouldn't have started.* My steps slowed. The rhythm faltered. Complaints swirled through my head: *My shoulder hurts. My back is tight. I want to get home.*

As I hunched forward into the wind and rain, I felt the battle more than heard it. It settled like a weight in my legs. Then awareness pulled my shoulders back. I heard the affirmation in my mind. *I am here and I am walking. I am here and I can do this. Yes, I can. Yes, I can.* The words pushed aside protests and complaints. They broke the trance of mindless babble. The chant began to match the rhythm of my steps until it condensed into a single word: *Yes!* I affirmed with each footstep. *Yes . . . Yes . . . Yes.* By the time I reached home, I had crossed a border. I had entered a new state of mind.

Day after day I return to the border. I step outside the door of my home and confront the hurdles on my walking path: *I don't have time. It's cold. It's hot. I'm tired.*

Anyone who walks regularly is familiar with the journey. No matter whether you walk alone or in a group, on treadmills or sidewalks or trails, you've stumbled over mental obstacles in your path. You've heard the hecklers who line the route. Summer, winter, rain, or shine, they wait beside the path. They hurl "to-dos" and "should-have-dones" in taunts that slow your step. Sometimes they even turn you back. But walkers who learn to silence these distractors travel to invigorating vistas. They reach inspiring heights. The peaks before us are hidden from view until we clear the fog in our own heads.

All too often we approach exercise as just another task— maybe even a burden. We do it because we know we should. "Stress walking," some folks have labeled it as they dash off to battle calories and advancing years with frantic lunch-hour sprints. Perhaps you're familiar with the pattern. You go on automatic, pushing through the paces of exercise while thinking about other things. You return from a thirty-minute walk with urgent memos swirling in your head. Even Henry David Thoreau, living in retreat at Walden Pond in the 1800s, recognized the hazard. "I am alarmed when it happens that I have walked a mile into the woods bodily, without getting there in spirit," he wrote. "The thought of some work will run in my head, and I am not where my body is,—I am out of my senses. In my walks I would fain return to my senses."[1]

The joyous connection that returns us to our senses occurs when body and mind fall into step together. It's as if we suddenly use two eyes instead of one to focus on a goal. Focus restores perspective. It transforms fitness walks into retreats of renewal and realignment. Focus guides us safely past the distractions that detour us from a path of well-being for body, mind, and soul.

Focus elevates ordinary walkers to the level of spiritual "saunterers," as Thoreau found on his meditative walks through the Massachusetts countryside. He credits the religious pilgrims of the Middle Ages for giving rise to the word.[2] Walkers who undertook pilgrimages to the Holy

Land, *la Sainte Terre*, came to be known as *Sainte-Terrers*. Not every walker reaches holy lands, Thoreau cautioned. Those who do are saunterers—not idle wanderers, as the modern word suggests, but purposeful travelers with a clear goal in mind. Travelers who leave familiar routes and routines to pursue a larger goal.

Surely, any expedition that leads to a greater sense of wholeness must be a pilgrimage to holy lands. Anyone who journeys toward spiritual and physical well-being earns the name of *Sainte-Terrer*. The pilgrimage on which I set forth as a walker urged me ahead at a brisk aerobic pace. It pushed me past fears I'd adopted long ago about getting hurt, getting dirty, or getting in trouble by letting my body run wild. Then, as the rhythm of walking teamed up with focus, I found a unity of movement that strengthened all of me. I became a "spirited walker."

## A STEP IN THE RIGHT DIRECTION

Millions of people already walk for fitness and health. The number surges with every study that delivers fresh evidence of walking's healthy contribution to everything from weight loss to memory improvement. We buy treadmills, pedometers, and heart monitors. We memorize cholesterol levels and aerobic heart rates. It's all a step in the right direction, but without focus, exercise walking loses much of its potency. By aligning the energies of muscles and mind, you make exercise more fun, more efficient, and more effective.

Simply following an exercise program, no matter what it is, can improve how you feel about yourself. It demonstrates that you are in charge of your life and are willing to act on your own behalf. Exercise translates beliefs into action—no wonder research confirms that regular exercise bolsters self-esteem! And when physical workouts team up with mental intention, the benefits increase.

No matter how fast or how far you walk, no matter what your goals or fitness level, the steps that transform exercise walking into a spirited, whole-body workout begin right where you are:

*Make a Move:* Spirited walking begins with the simple act of walking and with the recognition that walking has many parallels to life. Walkers move forward, take steps, go toward something. Walking is changing position, getting from one place to another. Whether you step around the kitchen table or trek across the country, the action changes your perspective. It offers a fresh point of view.

*Take a Chance:* Spirited walking is walking that pushes you out of your comfort zone. It feeds on curiosity and challenge. Try a new route or a different schedule. Join a walking group. When you step out of your comfort zone, past well-known patterns and paths, you venture into unexplored territory. The newness heightens your senses. You walk a trail toward self-awareness that takes exercise beyond heart rates and calorie burning.

*Get an Attitude:* Spirited walking is walking with awareness. Pay attention to how you talk to yourself when you exercise. The words you use reflect an attitude that is more

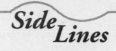
## Side Lines

### COMPOUNDING INTEREST AND YIELD

On days when you wonder why you make the effort to squeeze in exercise workouts for your body and your mind, consider the benefits. From peace of mind to self-esteem, from a longer life to a slimmer waist, the steps you take with a program of regular exercise and meditation can lead to paths of healing that modern researchers have traveled eagerly in recent years. New findings emerge almost daily in newscasts, offering fresh evidence of the far-reaching benefits of both walking and meditation. Put them together and the impact is strong medicine. Full health springs from a dynamic harmony of body and mind. Only then can we explore our potential for physical, emotional, and spiritual well-being.[3]

### WALKING BENEFITS

- Lowers blood pressure for people with elevated levels
- Improves cholesterol profiles by elevating good cholesterol
- Builds bone strength and decreases risk of osteoporosis
- Helps burn excess body fat and reduce weight
- Increases cardiovascular fitness
- Combats daily stress and anxiety
- Reduces severity of depression

- Eases chronic low-back pain

- Increases longevity

- Improves mood and mental performance

- Boosts the body's natural immune system

## MEDITATION BENEFITS

- Improves sleep patterns and reduces insomnia

- Reduces symptoms of depression and anxiety

- Assists in reducing allergy symptoms

- Provides relief from asthma

- Reduces number and intensity of migraines

- Lowers blood pressure for people with high levels

- Boosts the body's natural immune system

- Eases severity of PMS symptoms

- Reduces stress and stress-related illnesses

- Brings balance to high-pressure lives

important than where you walk, when you walk, and how fast or how far you travel. You carry this attitude with you wherever you go—whether you are on an athletic track, a city sidewalk, or a mountain trail.

*Go for More:* Spirited walking is walking that reflects a willingness to seek more from exercise. Try something different. Speed up your walking pace slightly. Extend your route a bit. Ask more than usual of yourself. In exchange, you'll get a workout that provides a metaphor. When you step forward boldly into a world of energetic movement, you set off on an exploration that will open doors in other parts of your life as well.

Because the body, mind, and soul are intricately connected, like the contents of a single cell, the movement of one part impacts another. Any change affects the whole. If you move a foot, the action pulses through all of you. Rearrange a thought, swallow an opinion, or uphold a belief, and the body reacts. Ultimately, those responses shape the way we feel about ourselves and how we view the world.

It could not be otherwise, maintains body-mind champion Deepak Chopra. "Your body is not just a shell or walking life-support system," he says. "It is your self intimately clothed in matter. Getting back in touch with this intimacy is very reassuring and delightful, particularly for people who have given up on exercise and become virtual strangers to their bodies."[4] If you're ready to strike up a reacquaintance, Chopra suggests thirty minutes of brisk walking daily as part of his prescription for healthy living and spiritual well-being.

When you begin to think of walking as more than an obligation, attitudes shift. You become conscious of metaphors that impact your life, your relationships, your self-image, your emotional health, and your spirituality. Fitness walkers are people who step out, step forward, make a move. So different from being stuck, stagnant, frozen in one position. *At least I'm out here walking,* you tell yourself when a winter wind blows up a flurry of excuses for turning back. *I'm moving forward. Moving toward my goal.* Each step brings an opportunity to confront the mental chatter that holds you back. Each step offers a chance to connect with yourself and your surroundings. *I can do it. I can do it. Yes-I-Can,* you chant to drown out voices that nag you to slow down.

Each step brings you to a threshold of awareness, focus, and choice. Will you continue to the corner or turn back here? Will you stop with fifteen minutes of walking, in spite of your goal to do twenty? Will you choose the words that guide your decision, or will you let your route be determined by the automatic responses that bounce through your brain without a sense of focus or destination?

Each question brings you to this moment. Just *hearing* the questions frees you from automatic responses. You are in control. When you choose to continue, you choose to focus on your movement and your goals rather than drifting into the mental distraction of shopping lists or relationship blunders. You stay connected to the present. That clear, conscious contact with the present is sometimes called awareness, or mindfulness—or even meditation.

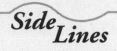

### GOING ON LOCATION

Is it possible to repeat a mantra while watching the "Wait" light flash above the crosswalk at the corner of the street? Can you keep your focus when a bus roars past? Is it safe to pay attention to your breath while you stride along the shoulder of a road? Do you need a quiet park or an athletic track in order to practice active walking meditation?

Any place where you can walk safely, you can walk safely with focus and intention. In fact, active meditation will heighten your awareness. The chances of being surprised by a bicyclist or Rollerblader whirling past are much greater when you walk and talk with a friend than when you walk alone, paying careful attention to your steps, your breath, or your self-talk. When you walk in silence, as a meditation, your senses are more alert. You hear sounds more quickly and notice movements out of the corner of your eye. Still, the right route can assist you in getting the most from both the walk and the meditation.

*Choose a flat, smooth walking course:* Start with a route that will not challenge you with steep hills or other physical barriers. Your goal is to find a path that lets you walk uninterrupted for as long as possible. If you live near a high school or college, try walking on the track at a time of day when it is not heavily used. Certainly, athletes learn to achieve focus and mindfulness in the midst of roaring fans and distracting competitors, but a relatively quiet environment facilitates the practice of mindfulness in the beginning.

*Take convenience over scenery:* If possible, select a location for your walking workouts that is convenient to your home or work so that it is easy to make active meditation part of your daily schedule. Scenic paths contribute greatly to walking pleasure, but only if they are easy to reach. Sometimes it's better to save a favorite walk in the country or beside the river for weekends unless you can make it part of your regular travel pattern.

*Seek firm footing:* Paved, graveled, or bark mulch surfaces let you set a brisk pace and maintain it safely. Uneven surfaces can disrupt the steady rhythm you want to establish with your movements. If possible, minimize the time spent on busy streets where your pattern will be interrupted by curbs and traffic lights at the end of each block. Remember to walk facing traffic if your route takes you through areas where there are no sidewalks.

*Put personal safety first:* Choose a walking route where you feel safe. For me, that route is in my neighborhood. Sometimes, when I want a change of scenery, I drive to a park where I walk beside the river. Because I usually walk alone, I go only during daylight hours and walk only in areas where other people are also exercising or working. If you would not feel safe alone, find a walking partner who is willing to accompany you in silence.

In many areas, community park and recreation departments, senior centers, and YMCAs sponsor regular walking groups. Groups create safety and energy, making it easier to maintain a walking program. Look for groups that strive for an aerobic pace. When the focus is on walking rather than chatting, you'll be able to keep your attention on walking with awareness.

## STEP TO THE INSIDE

Mention meditation and the first image that emerges for most of us is of someone sitting on a cushion in a quiet room. Traditional meditation techniques teach students to focus on the breath, gaze at a candle flame, or repeat a sacred word in order to clear the mind of distracting thoughts. Typically, we regard meditation as stillness for both body and mind. But that definition stifles the range and power of mindfulness.

Joan Borysenko, cofounder of the Mind-Body Medical Institute of Harvard Medical School, and author of several landmark books on mind-body connections, defines meditation as "any activity that keeps the attention pleasantly anchored in the present moment."[5] As modern research confirms the value of meditation in healing and physical well-being, new methods of mental centering have gained recognition. Prayers, poems, affirmations, or simply counting are espoused as useful tools for escaping stressful thought cycles that disrupt peace of mind. Yoga and forms of the martial arts also stabilize body and mind with a unifying focus.

But athletes meditate, too. No significant physical achievement is possible unless the athlete focuses clearly on a goal and believes that it is possible—a combination of physical, mental, and spiritual energy. I had never imagined this method of meditation in my years of sedentary "Om-ing." In fact, aerobic meditation seemed like a contradiction in terms until I stepped onto a path of personal discovery as a fitness walker.

Sometimes I find that the pairing of daily walks with the mental repetition of words or images produces a harmony of movement that flows through me with a resonance author Thomas Moore would call "enchantment." Moore maintains that our souls have "an absolute, unforgiving need for regular excursions into enchantment . . . like the body needs food and the mind needs thought."[6] Zen Buddhism acknowledges those moments of connection as "satori"—a melding of body, mind, and spirit that offers a fleeting sense of enlightenment, of oneness with nature and all life. Psychologists identify a human longing for "peak experiences" that infuse us with wonder and oneness. Athletes talk of being "in the zone" at times when purpose and motion are so clearly lined up that they feel invincible.

Each identifies an experience of congruency that exists only in the present moment. No mental hecklers. No past. No future. No lists of things to do. Just here. Just now. In other words, a state of meditation. Probably you recognize the feeling. Peak moments of clarity and connection remind us how it feels to be fully alive. These moments serve as private compass points as we travel toward physical and spiritual well-being.

## REGAINING CONSCIOUSNESS

It's always tempting simply to "space out" on a walk—to let the thoughts meander willy-nilly while we take a mental rest. Instead of rest, we often end up chasing loose ends and dodging arrows. The wonderful irony of conscious exercise is that by giving the mind a steady focus, you get the rest you seek. Studies show that walkers who simply repeat "in" and "out" with each breath reach a state of relaxation much faster than walkers who use no mental focus.[7]

But what about your weekly walk with a friend? The nightly stroll with the dog? And what of Sunday saunters by the river to watch the seasons change? Do those steps count as conscious exercise? Conscious exercise asks that you do one thing at a time. Walk with awareness and mindfulness. If your focus is on nurturing a friendship, social walking serves that need. If your hobby is spotting the nests of gray herons, a nature stroll by the river brings enormous satisfaction. But in terms of mental relaxation and spiritual connection, you travel farther if you don't divide your attention. Peace of mind results from mindfulness, from being fully aware and present in the moment—the opposite of distracted and adrift.

For walkers, the route to conscious exercise begins with a willingness to step out of your ruts. Take a walk alone instead of with the neighbor. Walk faster or longer. Ask more than usual of yourself—not so much that you put yourself at risk of physical strain or injury, but enough that you can't slide through the workout on automatic. Sooner or later you'll stumble over the roadblocks in your head. You will hear the voices that whine: *I'm tired. I'm bored. Isn't this enough? How important is this anyway? I feel silly walking alone.* At this moment, you face the same challenge that all meditators meet: side-talk in the mind. If you've ever meditated or used relaxation techniques, you're familiar with the process. A phrase from the disagreement at breakfast bounces up to disrupt your peace of mind. An image of the overflowing recycle bin in the garage pushes a mantra aside.

In both sitting and moving forms of meditation, mental-focusing tools help us silence protests and distractions. Now, if the smoke detector goes off during meditation, no one would advocate pushing aside the information. The same is true for a physical message that warns a walker of risk or injury. But most often the physical sensations that distract us arise out of habits and automatic mental patterns. As words of complaint or boredom surface, they mirror our responses in other areas of life. *What's the big deal?* you shrug as you flip on the television and abandon a resolution to catch up on some reading tonight.

Conscious walking, or spirited walking, lets you practice staying on track. Finishing the course. Focus provides a mental walking stick—something to lean on when the going gets tough. The metaphors bring an enriching addition to the physical benefits of regular exercise walking. They expand it beyond muscle tone and heart rates to connect the physical with the power and energy of our beliefs. Walking becomes both spiritually rewarding and physically refreshing as you open to a profound sense of connection with yourself and with the energy of life that surrounds you.

# From Sole to Soul . . .

*To* guide your journey into mindful walking, each chapter of *The Spirited Walker* offers suggested exercises. They outline a route to physical and spiritual well-being that is both playful and practical. Some of the exercises focus on aerobic fitness. Some derive from meditation. Some are just fun. All of them help you keep moving forward in a regular practice of spirited walking. Try them out to find activities that assist you in creating your own path toward physical and spiritual fitness. Expand them and change them with words that have significance to you.

Most of these exercises are designed to be done in silence, whether you are alone or with companions. If you never have time alone, this is an opportunity to claim a few quiet minutes of your own. If walking is your way to connect with friends, this is a chance to try something new together. Spend ten or fifteen minutes of warm-up at the start of each walk catching up. Then walk together silently for fifteen or twenty minutes while you experiment with the mental tools introduced in the exercise. Share your experience at the end of that period with some cool-down conversation. Group energy can boost your effort and your motivation.

Most of the workouts suggested in the *From Sole to Soul* section of each chapter can be completed in a thirty-minute period. If you have more than thirty minutes and feel physically prepared for a longer workout, increase the number of repetitions that you do or extend the time increments. If you're not physically ready for thirty minutes of walking, many of the exercises can be adapted to shorter times by reducing the repetitions. Most are flexible enough to be done in segments on walks of any length.

Each exercise introduces mental and physical skills that can increase the enjoyment and effectiveness of your fitness walks. Some are intended to motivate you. Some will push you to work a bit harder. As your workouts lead to increased endurance, strength, and commitment in meeting physical goals, these attitudes will spill over into other areas of your life and into the way you feel about yourself. Self-respect soars as you respect your body, your spirit, and your values with exercise that engages all of you.

*Shall We Waltz?:* Give yourself at least thirty minutes for this exercise. Allow five to ten minutes of easy walking to warm up and get the kinks out of your muscles. Now assume a comfortable walking gait, bend your arms at the elbows, and begin to swing them with each step. Try to maintain a ninety-degree angle in your arms so that your hands skim along your sides at waist level, swinging in an easy rhythm with your steps.

As you walk, keep your body erect, head up, and your eyes slightly down, focused on the path or street ahead of you. Mentally, begin to repeat these words in rhythm with each step and arm swing: *I am here. I am here.* One word per step.

This sounds pretty easy, and it is. You may find, however, that your tendency is to let yourself slip into a pattern of *I-am-here-pause, I-am-here-pause,* creating a four-beat rhythm. When this happens, you know that your attention has drifted. Instead, try to maintain a three-beat pattern, so that you are saying "I" on opposite sides of the body with each repetition. If the rhythm seems awkward, try playing the *Blue Danube Waltz* in the background. The three-beat measure is waltz rhythm. By setting your words to a waltz melody, you may dance through your workout more gracefully.

Speed doesn't matter right now. Walk as briskly as is comfortable for you while keeping your focus on the coordination of arms and words. By repeating a phrase, you create a focus that blocks out interfering thoughts, problems, and concerns. By alternating the rhythm in the three-beat pattern, you are creating a mind-body link that forces you to focus on what you are doing and thinking right now, as you walk. For most of us, the three-beat pattern is less familiar than a good old four-beat march. It takes more focus to maintain it.

Check your watch when you begin the active meditation and continue repeating *I am here* for ten to fifteen minutes. When you find your mind wandering, simply return to the phrase and the repetition. If you suddenly notice that your pattern has changed so that you are always saying "I" and "here" when your right arm swings forward, you will know that your focus has drifted and that your body has moved into a four-beat pattern. Bring yourself back to the three-beat rhythm and continue. If you want to stay with the phrase for longer than fifteen minutes, go ahead. Before you return to the routines of your day, take a few minutes to walk slowly and cool down. This is a great time to say a mental thank-you for things that support and enrich your life. Give thanks for successes and achievements. For opportunities. For a healthy body. Or for the people you treasure.

Try this exercise three or four different times to see if it gets easier for you to maintain the three-beat pattern as you walk. If it seems useful, you may want to create additional three-beat phrases of your own. Experiment with "Yes-I-can, yes-I-can," and "I-give-thanks, I-give-thanks." You'll soon be waltzing to your own rhythm.

# CHAPTER 2

~

# *On Your Mark*

## HOW FAR? HOW FAST? HOW OFTEN?

When a 1971 transit strike in Philadelphia halted the bus service that carried banker Mary Walker to her downtown office, she responded by doing what you'd expect from someone with her last name. She traveled seven miles to the bank on foot and then reversed the route to get home. "I enjoy walking," she says, shrugging off the notion that she did anything unusual. As the strike dragged on, the fifty-seven-year-old business woman discovered that walking paid dividends. When public transport returned to city streets, Mary stayed on the sidewalk. By then, she'd come to view the daily walks as a good investment in health and well-being.

Twenty-five years later, Mary hasn't changed her opinion. At eighty-two, she continues to walk, and to work. Following her mandatory retirement at age seventy, she was invited by her employer to stay on the job as a full-time, temporary employee of the bank. These days, she rides a train to the office. But from April to October, she walks home after work on a familiar route along the Schuylkill River. She covers the distance in about two and a half hours, maintaining a pace that averages a mile in twenty minutes. "The time varies, depending on if I stop to look at the river," she says. "It's such a beautiful walk."

Necessity prodded Mary into her walking habit, but today her motivation comes from the benefits that accompany her steps. After a day of interactions with people, she values a quiet time when she can release mental and physical stress. Until a reporter from the *Philadelphia Inquirer* expressed amazement that a woman in her eighties routinely walked seven miles a day, Mary had never measured the route. "I didn't care," she says. "I walk because I love it. Walking gives me a chance to meditate. It's good for the soul and quiets the mind. By the time I get home, all the little problems of the day have evaporated."[1]

Fortunately, you don't need to walk seven miles at a stretch to reap mental and physical benefits. Standard fitness guidelines recommend thirty minutes of moderately vigorous exercise three or four times a week to reduce risk of stroke or heart disease, diabetes, high blood pressure, osteoporosis, and colon cancer. But the U.S. surgeon general has

21

determined that those standards permit flexibility. Less strenuous activity of a longer duration provides about the same health benefits, according to a 1996 report by the Centers for Disease Control and the President's Council on Physical Fitness and Sports.[2] For example, a daily walk, at a pace of about two miles in thirty minutes, brings significant health benefits.

Mental health professionals report that just ten minutes of fast walking can promote mental alertness and reduce emotional stress. And a brisk ten-minute walk in the afternoon has been shown to boost energy levels longer than a candy bar.[3] Keep moving for a mile at a pulse-raising pace and you'll burn from seventy-five to more than one hundred calories, depending on your weight. In addition, you'll elevate your mood. When you pick up the length and frequency of walks, benefits expand, building muscle strength, endurance, bone density, and emotional well-being.

With all this opportunity at your feet, what are you waiting for? Getting yourself moving in the direction of whole-body walking doesn't require a lot of gear or preparation. All you really need is motivation—something that gets you started, the way a transit strike put Mary Walker in motion. If you are one of the millions of people who already walk for exercise, you've taken the first steps. Now you're ready to expand the skills you have. If fitness walking is not part of your current exercise routine, you'll find guidelines for getting started in this chapter. As you establish a regular walking practice, you'll learn to make mental awareness a part of your workouts. Awareness transforms routine walks into spirited walks. It teaches you to exercise consciously, in a way that doubles the benefits you accrue. Walking workouts fortify you physically, emotionally, and spiritually for full participation in a vibrant, healthy life.

While the suggested exercises in each chapter and the experiences of walkers you'll meet throughout the book provide tips for increasing the value of your walks, just remember that an approach that works for me or for another person may not suit you. As a journalist, I'm a professional "info-maniac"—I want to know my heart rate, distance, and how many calories I've burned. One of my regular walking companions never measures his pulse or his pace. Morning walks prepare me to face the day. Mary Walker finds an evening workout the perfect way to release office stress and reconnect with herself and with nature.

While discovering your preferences, experiment with suggested ways to hold your arms, your head, your torso. Become aware of how you move your body. Take your pulse one day and not the next. Try all the exercises. Too often we create enormous hurdles for ourselves by transforming suggestions into "rules" when we are learning new skills. Keep your focus on the goal of exploring new paths to physical and spiritual fitness.

## HOW FAR? HOW FAST? HOW OFTEN?

Walking can be a spiritual, meditative practice at any speed. Students of Eastern spiritual approaches often combine mental focusing techniques with slow meditative walking. The goal of spirited walking, however, is a walking practice that provides a cardiovascular workout as well as a mental one. When you put the physical effort of aerobic exercise together with mental awareness, workouts flood both body and mind with fresh air and fresh attitudes.

"Once you start walking, you'll discover the other reasons, such as what you feel in your body and mind during and after a great walk," confirms Kathy Smith, fitness video producer and enthusiastic walker.[4] "As you focus on the techniques and sensations of fast walking, the things that were driving you crazy a half-hour earlier slowly slip out of your mind."

*How Far?:* Let fitness be your guide. Make it your goal to walk for at least thirty minutes, including five to six minutes of warm-up and cooldown on each end and twenty minutes of aerobic effort in the middle. Another ten minutes of gentle stretching when you finish brings flexibility to your workout and becomes increasingly important as your walks gain intensity.

*How Fast?:* An average starting pace for healthy walkers falls between 2.5 and 3.5 miles per hour—a mile in twenty-four to seventeen minutes. Brisk walking is commonly defined as 3.5 to 4 miles per hour. But the key to spirited walking is not so much how fast you move as how fast your heart beats. Set a pace that pumps up your heart rate and your breathing. Take your pulse frequently in the beginning. Strive for a speed that gives you an aerobic heart rate, which is usually 70 to 85 percent of your maximum heart rate. Directions for establishing your target heart rate are included in this chapter.

*How Often?:* Three days a week, minimum. Add days if you want and if you are physically ready. Check with your doctor or a knowledgeable athletic trainer if you have questions about how much walking to attempt. Stay with it and you'll get hooked on the mental and physical boost that comes from active walking meditation. Walking is so body-friendly that you can do it every day without risk of injury. In fact, it's good for you. But don't be in a rush to expand your schedule, especially if you have been an irregular exerciser in the past.

Any exercise has value, of course. Working in the yard brings benefits. So does taking the stairs instead of the elevator or walking to the bank on your lunch hour. But the kind of walking that builds cardiovascular strength and mental control asks for a commitment. Walk regularly. Walk fast enough that your breathing becomes slightly heavy. That's when you'll encounter the challenges that give your mind a workout, too. Resistance shows up on every walk I take, and often more than once. It's the voice that thinks this is too much work. It's the urge to turn around and cut a workout short. It's the temptation to postpone a walk until the weather gets better or the holidays are over.

Confronting that resistance requires a partnership of mental and physical effort. You already possess a powerful mental tool if you're willing to use it. It's the skill that California State University psychologist Robert E. Thayer calls "cognitive override."[5] This means simply that you call for the boss whenever your commitment wobbles. Square your shoulders and speak in a firm voice to the detractors in your head. "Yes, yes, yes," you say. "I'd love to eat a cookie and stay inside to finish this project, but I know that I'll feel better if I get my exercise." Knowing that exercise improves mood and energy helps you "override" temptations and make holistic choices.

If you've struggled with a regular exercise program in the past, start cautiously in committing yourself to a walking schedule. Consider walking once a week with a regular walking group. Joining a group can help you establish a routine. Supplement the group by walking alone or with a partner two more days each week. Select a location and a time of day, and then stick to it all week. The fewer decisions you have to make before you put on your walking shoes, the better.

As you add days, build variety into the routes and the intensity of your walks. Go to the high school track. Look for a course that offers a hill. You'll strengthen different muscles and bypass the burnout that can arise when you repeat the same steps day after day. If you're walking five or six days a week, rotate fast strenuous walks with outings that are longer but at a slower pace. As part of that variety, put your feet up and give yourself a rest once in a while.

## In Pace with Wellness

To exercise at a pace and intensity that produce an aerobic workout, you'll need to know your target heart range— the pulse rate that you should "aim" for to achieve many of the health and fitness benefits of exercise.

You can figure out your target heart range by subtracting your age from 220. The result is considered a maximum heart rate for your age. Get out a calculator and multiply your maximum by 60 percent. Write down the answer. Multiply the same starting number by 85 percent. These two figures indicate the bottom and top of a training heart range for the average person of your age. If you are fit, aim for the higher end of your target range. If you're a little out of shape, stay on the low end at first. For most people, workouts that keep within 70 to 80 percent of target heart rate for twenty to thirty minutes bring safe and efficient aerobic benefits.

Monitor your heart rate by counting your pulse on your neck or wrist for ten seconds, beginning with zero as your first number. Multiply by six to get the number of beats per minute. Take your pulse often as you establish an aerobic walking speed. When you feel you are exercising at an aerobic level, pause for ten seconds and take your pulse. Are you within the target heart range? If your heart rate is lower than the target, increase your effort. If you've soared above 85 percent, slow down. Your pulse rate during exercise measures your body's fitness and readiness to handle stress. As fitness improves, you will be able to increase your speed gradually and remain in the target heart range.

Beginning walkers usually have no difficulty reaching target heart rates, but as fitness levels increase it takes more effort to sustain the same range for twenty minutes. Picking up the pace and adding a vigorous arm swing are two ways to elevate pulse rate and increase the aerobic benefits of walking. An inexpensive digital watch with numbers that are easy to read can help you monitor heart rate and walking speed. Use the watch to set goals and provide motivation. How long does it take you today to walk from your

## TARGET HEART RATES FOR AEROBIC EXERCISE[6]

| Age | Maximum Beats per Minute | 60% (10 sec) | | 70% (10 sec) | | 85% (10 sec) | |
|-----|------|-----|--------|-----|---------|-----|---------|
| 20 | 200 | 120 | (19-20) | 140 | (23) | 170 | (28) |
| 25 | 195 | 117 | (19) | 137 | (23) | 166 | (28) |
| 30 | 190 | 114 | (18-19) | 133 | (22) | 162 | (26-27) |
| 35 | 185 | 111 | (18) | 130 | (21) | 157 | (26) |
| 40 | 180 | 108 | (18) | 126 | (21) | 153 | (26) |
| 45 | 175 | 105 | (17-18) | 123 | (20-21) | 149 | (25) |
| 50 | 170 | 102 | (17-18) | 119 | (20) | 145 | (24-25) |
| 55 | 165 | 99 | (17) | 116 | (19-20) | 140 | (23-24) |
| 60 | 160 | 96 | (16-17) | 112 | (19) | 136 | (23-24) |
| 65 | 155 | 93 | (16) | 109 | (18) | 132 | (22-23) |
| 70 | 150 | 90 | (15-16) | 105 | (17-18) | 128 | (22-23) |
| 75 | 145 | 87 | (14-16) | 101 | (16-17) | 123 | (20-22) |

house to the intersection with the traffic light? How long to walk from the recreation center in the park to the tennis courts in the north corner? How long from the tennis courts to the drinking fountain? Pick a goal and time yourself whenever you walk that route. Take your pulse when you reach each destination.

People with limitations that prevent getting pulse rates into the 70 to 80 percent range can achieve the same physical benefits by walking longer. The American College of Sports Medicine advises that you need ninety minutes of sustained exercise to produce aerobic fitness when you walk at 60 percent of maximum heart rate.[7] At 85 percent of maximum, you get the same results in thirty minutes. So in terms of efficiency, it makes sense to work on increasing the speed and intensity of your steps.

Occasionally I encounter people in walking classes who have trouble locating a pulse point or who simply hate to bother. Several studies suggest that you don't need to. Check your perception instead. When exercisers are asked to rate exertion on a scale from "very, very light" to "very, very hard," most identify their appropriate aerobic level as "somewhat hard."[8] If you are breathing hard but not gasping and have reached a point of exertion that you'd call "somewhat hard," take your pulse to check your accuracy. If you've reached your target, maintain that level for twenty minutes. Before long, you'll come to recognize your aerobic workout level by the whining in your head: *This is hard. I don't feel like doing this anymore. What time is it, anyway?* You'll discover that exercise that delivers optimum aerobic benefits also gives a workout to the mind and spirit. You can train yourself to be aware of mental chatter and make active, informed choices about where you want to place your focus.

When you learn to merge mental focus and physical effort, fitness walking becomes spirited walking. That's the point at which you'll begin to "make the connection" to joy and self-acceptance that Oprah Winfrey discovered through a daily exercise program. As she learned to make wise choices, she connected with inner resources she had not known. "It was delightful, this new feeling of accomplishment brought on by pure discipline and self-control. It was exciting. . . . I felt like an athlete," she says.[9] By monitoring heart rate and exertion for a while, you'll gain a clearer understanding of your own mental and physical resources and know how to move forward, setting safe goals for a spirited walking practice.

If you've decided that it's too much trouble to take your pulse at all, at least take time to consider the metaphor. Are there other places in your life where you are not willing to make the effort to get clear, accurate information? Perhaps you have a pattern of deceiving yourself about your level of effort and commitment. By choosing to ignore information, you may be putting yourself at risk of injury when you exercise. Certainly you are putting yourself at risk of disappointment.

## FOCUSED ON ACTION

"The difference between those who successfully achieve their dreams and those who remain frustrated is the ability to move from desire to action," maintains sport psychologist Shane Murphy.[10] If you picked up this book with dreams of becoming physically fit or of expanding opportunities for spiritual exploration, you need to get specific if you really want to achieve those outcomes. The road to making dreams come true is paved with stepping-stones. Effective goals spell out clear actions you will take. For a new walker, an action goal might be to buy a pair of walking shoes. Period. No mention of long-range results. Just completing the action brings a sense of achievement and accomplishment that keeps you moving toward your goal.

"Action goals energize us. Results goals
Murphy says, reciting a rule of thumb that er...
seven years of working with America's top amateur athletes
as chief psychologist to the U.S. Olympic Committee. It's
OK to want results. Just be sure you know how to get them.
When you set effective action goals, you experience success
with each workout. You create opportunities to congratulate yourself for taking positive action. The key is to focus
on the steps that will lead you to the goal.

You'll get off on solid footing with your spirited walking
program if you take a minute to consider the results that
you seek:

- Improved physical fitness?

- A longer life span?

- Weight loss?

- Quiet time alone?

- Workouts you can enjoy?

- Trimmer hips?

- An opportunity for meditation?

- Spiritual enrichment?

- Physical stamina?

- ~~Confidence to walk in a community fund-raiser?~~

- A sense of body-mind wholeness?

- A regular walking habit?

Aim at targets that are out of reach but not out of sight, Murphy advises in *The Achievement Zone,* a guide to mind-body skills for sports and daily life. Focus on daily and weekly goals that will guide you toward your target with clear, specific actions. Perhaps you decide to walk for thirty minutes three times a week. Now you have an action plan you can measure. Vague promises will get you nowhere, Murphy warns. A loose agreement to "do your best" is little more than an escape clause that frees you from making a real effort. Success requires a combination of mental commitment and physical action.

## AN INVIGORATING STEP

Physical action should be the easy part of a successful walking program. After all, you know how to walk already. Still, many of the people I see on my daily walks are missing out on many of the health and fitness benefits of walking. The vast majority of the people who walk for exercise err on the side of underexertion. They never sweat. They never breathe hard. They never ask their bodies to tolerate the discomfort that confirms they're actually putting some "work" in a walking "workout." As a result, they fool themselves about the aerobic benefits their walks provide.

Often it's their mental muscles that need stretching. They've simply never learned to see walking as an athletic activity. When I referred to walking as the most popular sport in America, an acquaintance looked at me quizzically. "Can you really call walking a sport?" he asked. You bet it's

# Side Lines

## GEARING UP FOR WALKING

Walking owes a lot of its popularity to its no-nonsense practicality. Compared to most sports, it's low risk and low maintenance. You can do it just about anywhere, and you don't need a lot of high-tech equipment. In fact, you don't really need anything different from what you might wear to a movie. Good shoes, comfortable clothing, and a wristwatch supply the basics.

*Shoes:* Certainly shoes are a walker's most important piece of equipment, and the most complex. With many styles available, it isn't always easy to know which one will be best for your feet and your workouts. Many walking shoes are designed for strolling, not for active aerobic walking. These sturdy shoes offer great support for sight-seeing or running errands but often do not provide adequate flexibility for walkers who want to move at a brisk pace. Test the flexibility of the sole by bending the shoe with your hands. You'll soon discover that some styles offer more movement in the ball of the foot. That's important when you pick up the pace of walking and push off with the toes.

Many fitness walkers opt for running shoes in order to get a light, flexible shoe. Here, too, you need to make a careful choice. Look at the heel. The thick flared heels of many running shoes can create imbalance for walkers. Because walkers hit the ground heel first, you want a shoe with shock absorption in the heel and a stable landing surface. Some run-walk shoe styles have a beveled heel so that you land on a flat surface. At most fitness-walking speeds, this isn't essential. At racing speeds, it can increase stability and heel-to-toe roll-through.

Choose a shoe that feels comfortable and gives you plenty of room around the toes. You want space to roll forward on the foot without jamming into the front of the shoe.

*Socks:* Take advantage of technology to make walking more comfortable and blister-free. Synthetic blends fit the foot more snugly than wool or all-cotton socks and provide wicking that carries moisture away from the skin to minimize rubbing.

*Wristwatch:* A simple digital watch from the drugstore can add motivation, evaluation, and satisfaction to your walking program. Look for a model with a few sporty options to increase its benefit as a tool that challenges and rewards you. The large, easy-to-read numbers of a digital watch make it easier to take ten-second pulse checks during your walks. Pick out a style that includes a stopwatch. Set it when you begin the twenty-minute aerobic segment of your workout and you won't have to remember exactly when you started. On other days, use the stopwatch to give yourself short speed drills. Or time how long it takes to walk a mile.

A few companies produce a "walking" or "pacer" model with an optional beep that you can program to match your walking pace. The pacer works like a metronome to keep your rhythm steady. It's a handy tool when you are trying to increase speed, but be aware that the sound can be annoying to other people. Be considerate and use it only when you are outdoors. With prices that start at about twenty-five dollars, a plastic sports watch is a valuable piece of walking equipment. Once you make your way through the instructions and learn to time your workouts, you'll start to feel like an athlete. As a bonus, most include an alarm-clock feature that can get you up and walking, even on vacation.

a sport! Anyone who thinks otherwise hasn't tried aerobic walking. Start walking like an athlete, and you'll discover new respect and a new range of motion in the simple movement pattern you've taken for granted most of your life.

Several years ago I stumbled into that challenging realization during a vacation trip to the Southwest. When I joined a group for a desert walking excursion, I found myself on a route to amazement. Setting the pace was a man whose brisk step took me by surprise. As he chatted comfortably about the landscape, I limped through the awkward rhythms of jog-a-little-walk-a-little just to stay at his side. My twenty-year age advantage and regular participation in aerobics classes didn't prepare me for the challenge that he presented by walking a twelve-minute mile. He moved with steady vigor and energy. By the time we completed a two-mile circuit, my side ached, my hips hurt, my shins cried out in pain. But even in the exhaustion, my mind bubbled with excitement. Until then, it hadn't occurred to me that walking could be aerobic exercise. With this new realization, I felt a surge of curiosity and challenge, the exhilaration of an explorer setting foot on uncharted shores. Along with desert scenery I'd glimpsed an expanded point of view. Walking came into focus as a sport, as different from hiking or strolling as Jazzercise is from ballet.

Because walking is so much a part of our lives, we don't pay much attention to it. As with breathing, or listening, we assume we know how to do it until we take a deep breath and pay closer attention. When you begin to walk with mental and physical awareness, you move toward something new. Just being willing to try something different—to walk faster, farther, quieter, or taller—sets you off on an adventure. It opens your mind to expanded possibilities and to exploration of the unknown.

"All walking is discovery," observed *New York Times* nature writer Hal Borland, whose essays reminded readers for thirty years to look with appreciation at the world around them. "On foot we take the time to see things whole."[11]

## STRIDE RIGHT

Start your adventure on the right foot physically by being conscious of posture and techniques that permit your body to move efficiently. Familiarity with the physical aspects of walking gives you a safe base on which to establish your own practice. By paying respectful attention to your physical abilities, your limitations, and your heart rate when you begin an exercise program, you prepare yourself to move forward in a manner that will bring success. Be aware, however, that "respectful attention" to your body does not mean settling for a halfhearted effort.

"Any change requires an initiatory period of discomfort, until the body adjusts to the new demand. You will experience this discomfort as you develop your talent; there is no way of getting around it," insists Dan Millman, the inspirational coach who wrote *The Way of the Peaceful Warrior.* Be patient and persistent and the discomfort will disappear as the body readjusts and accepts a new pattern. "The real journey, you see, is a journey within your own body."[12]

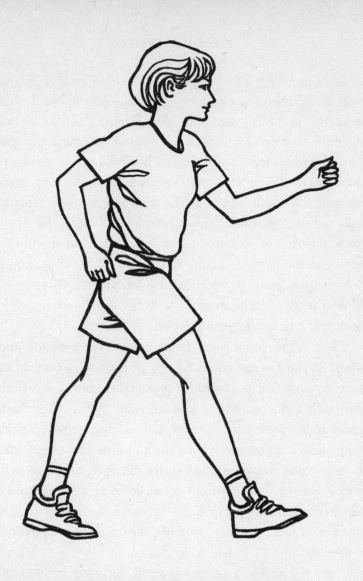

Good fitness walking posture holds the body tall with shoulders relaxed and spine straight. Eyes focus on the path ahead to keep the chin tucked. Arms swing actively at the sides. Lean forward slightly, keeping the body tall and erect so the lean begins at the ankle as if you are "falling" forward into each step. Maintain an easy stride length, pushing off with the toes to propel the body forward.

*Body Tall:* Imagine that your chest, shoulders, neck, and head are attached to cords that lift you gently. Hold your head erect and relax your shoulders. Tighten and tuck your buttocks slightly. You'll feel your spine lengthen and the base of your pelvis tip forward. This position protects the lower back. When you lean forward to walk, keep your body in a smooth line. Let the lean begin at the ankles, rather than the waist. Many people lead with the chest when they try to pick up speed. Soon the chin tips up in front and the buttocks push out behind. This can lead to a swayed back, putting stress on the lower torso. If you feel tension in your back after brisk walking, pay attention to posture the next time you exercise.

*Head High:* Keep your head erect, eyes forward and aimed at the ground about fifteen to twenty feet ahead of you. A visored cap assists in narrowing your vision and eliminating distractions. Focusing your eyes on the path ahead holds your head in a relaxed, upright position with chin tucked as you move forward and also encourages you to turn your mental focus inward. Peripheral vision will permit you to see movement on either side. Be mindful of personal safety and maintain a narrow range of focus only when you feel comfortable with the traffic and physical conditions.

*Arms Active:* For a warm-up stroll, let your arms swing freely at your sides, alternating with the legs. A good arm swing brings balance to your walk and increases circulation throughout the body. As you pick up the pace, bend the arms into a ninety-degree angle. Form soft, relaxed fists with your hands, and try to keep your arms close to your sides as they swing back and forth. Let your wrist and fore-arm lightly graze the hip with each swing.

*Heel First:* For a fluid walk, think of your feet as rockers. The ankle is the hinge. Land on your heel and roll forward to a smooth push-off with the toes. Keep your steps short. Overstriding creates a jerky walking style that wears you out. To walk faster, take more steps, not longer ones. The number of steps, or "turnover," determines how fast you go. Increasing turnover is the key to increasing speed.

*Breath Full:* Take deep breaths that go clear to the belly. Shallow breathing contributes to fatigue, muscle cramps, and side aches. Develop a full, smooth breathing rhythm to fuel your body with oxygen. When you find that you are breathing harder than you do normally, you are working your heart and lungs. You are also filling your cells with oxygen, which increases energy.

Many excellent books offer information about walking techniques and the physiology of aerobic exercise. Rather than duplicate those resources, this book focuses more on how you *think* when you walk. Take a look at a fitness-walking resource book for advice on questions you may encounter regarding form, pace, or training programs. Most public libraries will have several options. Good choices include *Prevention's Practical Encyclopedia of Walking for Health,* by Mark Bricklin and Maggie Spilner; *Walk Aerobics,* by Les Snowdon and Maggie Humphreys; and *Kathy Smith's WALKFIT for a Better Body,* by Kathy Smith with Susanna Levin. You'll find these and other suggestions in the resource section at the end of this book.

## MOVING TOWARD MEDITATION

As you set clear action goals and become attentive to the way you move when you walk, you embark on the mental exercise that accompanies spirited walking. "The objective of meditation is to gain control over your attention, clearing the mind and blocking out the stressors responsible for increased tension," says fitness researcher Werner Hoeger.[13] Spirited walking uses active focusing techniques as tools that hold the attention still rather than revisiting last night's dinner conversation or stewing over that comment your boss made three days ago. By concentrating on the immediate effort, the attention stays in the present. You begin to meditate.

"Focus your thoughts and your actions on one small aspect of the present, and you will create personal power," confirms Jerry Lynch, founder of the Tao Center for Human Performance. "Giving full attention to the present moment is energizing and enables you to control the current reality. You must be present in order to win."[14]

You may discover that walking by yourself helps you stay on course mentally as you make workouts a time of active meditation. If you find that walking with a partner creates greater safety or motivation for you, select companions who want to share the path in silence. Support one another by setting distance targets and agreeing not to talk during those segments of your walks. If you walk at compatible speeds, you'll be able to help each other maintain an aerobic pace. Walking alone, or with others in silence, gives you an opportunity to explore your own mental process, free from the distraction of other people's conversation or your own social expectations. It separates you for a few minutes from the demands that split contemporary lives into fragments with separate slots for work, play, meals, and meditation. In this quiet place, you create a moment of integration that promotes a healthy wholeness of muscles, mind, and spirit.

# From Sole to Soul . . .

*Goal Mining:* When you know clearly what you want, you've taken the first step toward getting it. The ability to identify a target gives you something to aim for. What motivated you to pick up this book? What did you hope to find? An exercise program? Inspiration? A way to enrich daily walks? A time-saving combination of exercise and meditation? When you know what you'd like to achieve, you have the information you need to begin moving toward a goal. Make an action agreement with yourself to take a step in that direction this week. Perhaps your agreement is to do the timed-mile exercise that follows so that you have information about your walking speed as a guide to setting progressive goals. Or you may agree to get out and walk for thirty minutes three times this week, focusing on good walking posture. Perhaps your agreement will be to walk in silence for a week to experience something new.

The important thing is to make an agreement that you can measure and that is appropriate for your present fitness level. Be respectful of all the other commitments in your day as you choose an action agreement that is realistic. By learning to set appropriate action goals, you learn to create success and bring a sense of accomplishment into your life.

Now, *write your action agreement on a sticky note and put it where you'll see it!* Try the refrigerator door or the bathroom mirror. It wouldn't hurt to put it in both places.

When you are trying to learn new habits or change the patterns of your day, it's helpful to have reminders. Later on, you won't need them. Your mind will have shifted to adopt the new pattern, and you'll be ready for the next step toward your goal. Review your action goals weekly as you experiment with active walking meditation. If you decide to keep the same goal for an additional week, rewrite it on a new sticky note so that your reminder is fresh and eye-catching.

Stay curious and willing to try new ideas until you find a schedule, a pace, and a walking style that invigorate your body and your spirit. Keep in mind that mental skills are really no different from physical ones; they improve with practice.

*Marking Time:* As a measure of your walking fitness level and a starting point for realistic goal setting, it's useful to know how long it takes you to walk a mile at a brisk but comfortable pace. This information will let you measure progress in your fitness and aerobic level as you move forward in a regular walking practice.

Schedule at least thirty minutes for this exercise and plan to go to a high school or college track where distance is easy to measure. If you can't get to a track, you can use a flat, one-mile course that has been measured and marked in a park or on a street you have driven. You'll also want a stopwatch or timer. On a standard outdoor track, one lap on the inside lane equals 440 yards or one-fourth mile. Some tracks measure 400 meters, a couple yards short of one-fourth mile but close enough to give you a good indication of your basic walking pace. As you move to outside lanes, each lap gets longer and you travel farther.

If you are a healthy, moderately active walker, you will probably complete a mile in fifteen to twenty minutes. If you consider yourself relatively inactive and don't feel ready to walk a full mile yet, cut the distance in half. A base time for a half-mile walk will be just as valuable. Remember, this exercise builds your information file; it is not a race.

Do a couple of easy warm-up laps when you get to the track. If you aren't used to walking on a track, this will give you an opportunity to get accustomed to the surface and the surroundings. Track etiquette asks that you walk in the outside lanes during warm-up and cooldown phases so that you leave the inside lanes clear for people who are doing timed workouts. After your warm-up, get a drink of water and limber up with a couple of very gentle stretches. Rotate shoulders, hips, and ankles to prepare them for an extended walk. Then move to the inside lane and start your watch.

Walk at a pace you think you'll be able to maintain for a mile, or for half a mile if that's the goal you have chosen. You want the pace to be steady and purposeful but not exhausting. If you find yourself battling mental objections as you walk, practice the waltz step you learned in the last chapter, affirming "I am here" or using your own three-word phrase. Stay focused on your goal. If you hit the final stretch with energy to spare, pick up the pace and finish strong.

Snap off your timer as you cross the finish line and take a few steps toward the outside edge of the track to clear the inside lanes. Pause to take a ten-second pulse check before you slow down. Is your heart rate within the target heart range for your age? Is it higher or lower than the target? Use that information to adjust your effort in the future.

Allow your heart rate to drop gradually by walking an easy cooldown lap. End the exercise with gentle stretches to relax the muscles you have stressed. How fast or slow you have walked doesn't matter. Jot down your time and your heart rate on your calendar or in a notebook when you get home. This information gives you a useful reference for the future.

*Elbow Action:* Try this exercise for two to three minutes any time you want to increase your walking speed and raise your heart rate. Be certain that you are thoroughly warmed up and moving at a smooth, easy pace before you swing into Elbow Action.

Pick a short target distance, maybe a block or half a lap on a track, and set off at a good fast clip. Review your posture as you move: body tall and upright, chin down, shoulders relaxed, arms bent and swinging at your side, buttocks tucked slightly to straighten your back. Push yourself to keep a brisk pace.

Now, without slowing down, draw your focus to your arms. Pick up the tempo of your arm swing. Most people are shocked to discover they can change the speed of their feet simply by swinging their arms. Let the arms set your speed for two or three minutes of intense movement and then check your posture. Are your shoulders still relaxed? Are your hands in soft fists? Work on speeding up without tightening up. Loose shoulders move much more efficiently than stiff ones.

Ultimately, the legs hold the power to set your pace. Fitness level determines how long you can maintain a speed. But a strong arm swing contributes energy to active aerobic walking. By focusing on the elbows for a few minutes when you feel your body slowing down, you can pump up the pace again. Use Elbow Action to trigger awareness of posture and to remind yourself that whole-body walking draws on the power available when every part of you is working together. Even your elbows contribute energy.

# CHAPTER 3

*Words for Walkers*

I Am Here and I Am Walking

After an hour on the road, we were eager to start walking when we reached the trailhead in the Santa Catalina Mountains outside Tucson. We lumbered out of the van, stiff from the early morning drive, and pulled on daypacks without conversation. We were still adjusting straps and smoothing on sunscreen as we fell into place behind our guide and began a three-mile descent into the canyon.

At the lead, Phyllis wove through a stand of fragrant pines and set a brisk pace that I followed automatically. The drive had numbed my senses. When she jumped suddenly to the side of the trail, a chain reaction bounced down the line of hikers and jerked us to alertness.

"Rattlesnake!" buzzed the person ahead of me.

"Rattlesnake," I hissed to the hiker behind.

Then we saw it—dark and dangerous in a sunny patch of mountain trail. No need for pulse checks at this point. I could feel my heart pounding in my throat.

Phyllis assessed the situation coolly. An experienced hiking guide who knew the routes and the risks of these slopes, she decided there was room for all of us on the abandoned road we were following. She urged us to move quietly along the edge of the path, leaving the snake undisturbed. My body buzzed with energy as I stepped forward, eyes locked on the black threat. A heady dose of survivalist adrenaline fueled my elation as I moved safely out of range. Instantly the aches and pains that had accompanied me out of the van at the trailhead disappeared. I felt ebullient and powerful.

The feeling lasted at least an hour, carrying me to the midway point of the hike. During a brief rest at the site of an abandoned miner's cabin, we snacked on trail mix and bran muffins while reliving our brush with danger and congratulating one another, as victors do, for our calm in the face of crisis. We chatted eagerly now, no longer a group of eight strangers brought together by a sign-up sheet at the resort where we were guests.

I was a novice hiker. But as a basically healthy woman, I expected to have no difficulty with the seven-mile hike described as a butterfly route—down one wing, a breather at the bottom and then a climb up the other. When I added

my name to the sign-up list, the greatest challenge seemed
to be the 6:30 A.M. departure time. Now, nourished by trail
mix and adrenaline, I felt invincible.

Before we'd tired of congratulatory reflection, Phyllis
stood and turned her gaze uphill. As we left the shade at the
bottom of the trail, the Arizona sun slapped us on the back.
Experienced hikers in the group pulled out sun hats and
neckerchiefs for protection. The route was steep, with only
sparse patches of shade. I leaned into the slope and felt the
heat of June coil up from the rocks beneath my feet. Very
quickly, the energy that had buoyed my steps into the
canyon evaporated. My legs felt heavy, my mouth dry. I
paused to sip water from the bottle in my pack and wondered if I had made a mistake. Self-doubts started nagging
at my mind. Did I take on too much with a day in the
mountains? Was I fit enough for a steady uphill climb?
What if I couldn't make it out of the canyon? Here, on an
organized hike with experienced leaders, there was no real
danger of being lost or left behind—only the danger of
being embarrassed, only the risk of failing to perform. Still,
the questions mounted. Reasoning has little influence on
self-doubt.

Within minutes, all I could hear in my head was complaint: *I'm hot. I'm tired. My legs ache. . . . I'm hot. I'm tired. I
can't do this. . . .* Over and over it went. Eventually, the
chant slowed my pace to a faltering stumble. Step-stop-
gasp. Step-stop-gasp. Each move became a battle. Finally
the sun burned through my resistance and lit a flame of
clarity in some far corner of my mind. I knew that I'd never
get out of the canyon on my own if I continued this litany.

Or if I did manage to survive, by some incredible stroke of personal strength and good fortune, I'd carry with me such dreadful memories of hiking that I'd never want to do it again.

There on a rocky uphill climb, I had stumbled upon a challenge. Not long before, in my work as a journalist, I'd watched a group of ordinary people take off their shoes and walk quite willingly across a hot bed of burning coals in a demonstration of mind over matter. They emerged uninjured and exultant at the end, giving credit to mental power. Now I seemed to be crossing hot coals of my own. I wondered if I, like the fire walkers I had seen, could complete a walk that would leave me joyful instead of scarred. I wondered if I could change the way I was feeling by changing the talk in my head.

In the shade of a scraggly oak, I considered the possibilities. When I began to climb again, I tried to reverse the words that dragged me down. *I am graceful,* I huffed, as I plodded up the slope. *I am strong. I am fit.* I wanted to feel at ease on the trail. Instead of the awkward, clumsy sense of myself I had at that moment, I wanted to feel strong and comfortable. I wanted to know that I could get to the top of the trail comfortably and enjoy it. But as I plodded up the hill, my thoughts returned stubbornly to the heat and my discomfort. My mind clung tenaciously to each complaint it could devise.

*I am graceful,* I insisted, as I trudged up the incline. *I am strong. I am healthy.* Slow and steady. One word per step. In the shade, I'd stop to catch my breath and bargain with myself: a drink of water when I reach the next tree. A massage when I get back. And so I continued, a hike of negotiation and affirmation that carried me at last to the van at the top of the trail. Eventually, it took me much further than I could have imagined. That day in the Santa Catalina Mountains signaled a significant turning point in my life. What emerged from the uphill battle of words and wills was an affirmation that challenged and motivated me. It signaled the start of a new relationship with myself.

*I am a graceful and active woman, at ease in a strong, healthy body,* I decided after trying out other versions of the affirmation. The words sounded awkward as I repeated them. Unnatural and untrue. But I liked the possibility of it. I liked the strength of it. Now, a dozen years later, the affirmation feels like a core truth in my life. The words have become a private signature, a phrase I chant to myself on trails and sidewalks when I begin to tire or doubt myself. The words dispelled childhood ghosts of clumsiness. They guided me to the discovery that a sense of spiritual connection and wholeness comes not only from the mind, the heart, the soul. It rises from the body as well.

## In the Beginning Was the Word

From the word *go,* walking often seems to be as much a verbal activity as a physical one. Just getting yourself to the door elicits a flurry of questions and protests. *Is there enough time for a walk? It's too cold. It's too hot. What about watering the garden? Shouldn't you go to the cleaners for your suit?*

# Side Lines

## TAPPING THE POWER OF SELF-TALK

When you want to make your walks a meditation, you will find that words and phrases help you keep your attention focused and present. That's what meditation really is. Many meditators use traditional words with spiritual origins as a mental focus for their thoughts. Frequently, these words refer to a divine source or power. But any word, sound, or phrase that seems meaningful to you can get you started on a practice of focused walking. Athletes often use words or phrases that affirm a mental or physical state they want to maintain. Let these suggestions of spiritual and secular meditation words stimulate your own creative choice of a mental walking companion:

- **Om:** Sanskrit word meaning "the beginning, the source"

- **Rama:** Sanskrit word meaning "to rejoice"

- **Hail Mary** or **Ave Maria:** from Catholicism

- **God, Holy Father, Lord Jesus:** from Christianity

- **Shalom:** Hebrew word meaning "peace"

- **Ham sah:** Sanskrit mantra said to echo the sound of inhaling and exhaling

- **Love**
- **Nature**
- **Relax**
- **Release**
- **Peace**
- **Let go**

- Focus
- Be here now
- Calm
- Breathe

Remember that meditation means staying present. You are in your body, aware of your movement and breath instead of letting aimless thoughts drag you around. Experiment with using an affirmative phrase to help you focus when you walk. The words you select can have spiritual significance for you, or they can be directed at the physical and mental state you want to achieve as you walk.

I am healthy and whole.
Strong and able
I give thanks.
Om mani padme hum
Thanks be to God.
God is love.
I am confident and capable.
I am moving with grace and ease.
I am one with all.
Thy will be done.
I am at peace.
Smooth and steady

If you'd like more examples of affirmations for daily living, you might look at *Creative Visualization,* by Shakti Gawain, or *Words That Heal,* by Douglas Bloch. For affirmations directed toward athletic performance as well as business and daily life, try *Thinking Body, Dancing Mind: TaoSports for Extraordinary Performance in Athletics, Business, and Life,* by Chungliang Al Huang and Jerry Lynch.

By the time you tie your walking shoes and shut the door behind you, you've cleared the hurdles of a mental steeplechase and demonstrated strong determination. But unless you've discovered an easy way to leave your brain on the doorstep, you're probably going to confront the same hurdles at every corner on your walk. Words are both the *challenge* and the *solution* for those who want to transform walks into meditative breaks from daily stresses.

"You are what you think," says Joe Henderson, an editor at *Runner's World* magazine. "And in sports, that can be either a blessing or a curse, depending on the quality of your thinking."[1]

Rather than fighting the words that distract or discourage, successful athletes and experienced meditators learn to replace them with words that keep the mind in the present moment. Meditators often use a word, a phrase, or sound, called a mantra, to quiet and focus the mind. In Sanskrit, the word *mantra* indicates a word or sacred formula that is offered as a prayer. In many meditation techniques, students repeat a mantra as a way of blocking out distracting thoughts and giving full attention to a spiritual concept. With practice, meditation teaches you to control your focus and free yourself from the automatic cycles of "shoulds" and "ought-tos" that bombard you all day long.

For walkers, a mantra can be any word that provides mental focus for walking meditation. Simply repeating "Yes, yes, yes" in rhythm with each step or each exhalation of breath can be a powerful mantra when you are feeling resistant or bogged down. "Right here, right now," has a similar power to keep your thoughts in the present. When you catch yourself thinking of buying a birthday present or getting the car serviced while you are walking, the affirmation that *I am here and I am walking,* gives you a gentle reminder to return to the present and to the words that keep you focused in the moment.

Affirmations are positive self-statements, words you can use to counteract negative self-talk. Affirmations state a goal, a way you want to feel or be. An affirmation is always stated as a fact and always in the present tense. Often, it begins with *I am. I am strong and powerful. I am prepared and relaxed. I am happy and confident.*

Think of affirmations as a kind of in-house advertising program. The more you hear the message, the more you believe it. After a while, it becomes a part of your life. You wonder how you got along without it. The message of an affirmation is stronger and more effective if you word it as if it is true right now. Instead of saying *I am becoming fit and healthy,* say, *I am fit and healthy.* Instead of *I try to do the best I can,* say, *I am doing the best I can,* or *I do my best and I accept myself.*

You will know when you've hit an emotional trigger point with your words. For me, a ripple of energy that raises goose bumps on my skin confirms that I've made contact with a central current in my life. Your signal may be similar, or perhaps you'll feel a rush of warmth on your cheeks, a buzz in your ears. Some people don't experience a physical response but know they've made a connection with truth when they sense a mental "aha." Depending on your own belief system and the words you use to describe your spiritual world, this reaction may signal connection with your own inner knowing, with your higher self, or with a spiritual power.

Walking deepens the effectiveness of affirmations and mantras by making the message cellular. Because body and mind are inseparable, a joyous harmony arises when words and walking fall into step within a workout. Brain patterns merge with body patterns. The rhythmic repetition of words and movement deepens mental relaxation and opens pathways of integration. Linus Mundy calls it "taking a stroll with your soul." Mundy wrote a pocket guide called *Prayer-Walking*,[2] which encourages walkers to establish a spiritual fitness program by reciting a passage of scripture, a prayer, or a poem while walking. Walking and prayer complement one another by leading us on journeys that are simultaneously internal and external, he says. Putting the words of prayer together with fitness walking in a regular workout schedule can strengthen our physical bodies and the relationship we have with ourselves, and it can also strengthen our connection with a spiritual power or higher consciousness.

## WORDS OF PRAISE AND POWER

The words that bring energy and focus to the walking workouts of a fifty-seven-year-old speech pathologist in New York City literally sing with hope and faith. As she exercises, the lyrics of hymns set a rhythm of praise in her brain.

"Oh, you brought me, yes, you brought me, from a mighty long way. Thank you, Jesus, thank you, Jesus," she sings to herself to set an upbeat pace that leaves casual joggers behind.[3] The words are more than a rhythmic mantra. They remind her to be grateful that she's able to walk at all.

In her late forties, Elton Richardson was diagnosed with a severe case of osteomalacia, adult rickets. The diet-related illness almost crippled her before it was reversed with massive doses of calcium and vitamin D. During her recovery, Elton decided to make regular exercise part of a healthier lifestyle. She joined a group of Sunday joggers in a Brooklyn park and took the first steps toward changing an image that had hobbled her since fourth grade when she shot up to her full five feet nine inches and began to view herself as a misfit.

"I thought I was the ugliest thing in the whole world," she says. "I had no self-confidence. I was the world's biggest klutz." Not surprisingly, she turned her attention to academic successes and avoided confrontation with the part of her that had caused so much embarrassment—a body that didn't fit. The diversion worked fine until disease forced a "use it or lose it" relationship.

First she jogged. Then she ran. She chalked up several marathons. Then, at fifty, she turned to walking and quickly reached her stride. As a competitive racewalker, she began setting American and world walking records. She picked up gold medals at every distance from 1,500 to 40,000 meters. Along the way, she also picked up a new attitude.

"I can do it," she affirms to herself when faced with a challenge in any corner of her life. "I can do it," she repeats when doubts appear.

"I am so happy," she says. "I know now that I can do things. It hasn't always been this way. I never set out to be a

57

champion; it just happened." Now she walks out of gratitude to God for the healing that produced her present level of physical and emotional strength. When she races, she sets her pace with prayers, chanting, "Thank you, Jesus," with each step. Sometimes she turns to a familiar Sunday school song. "Yes, Jesus loves me," she tells herself. The rhythm perks up her pace when energies start to sag; the message fills her with reassurance: "It reminds me that he is there and that he loves me. I am much more aware of my spiritual self. I have grown stronger spiritually."

Although she was initially seeking a way to restore physical health and flexibility, walking has reached into every area of her life and thought. She has learned that no matter what she sets out to do, it's going to go better with a clear head. "If your head is full of doubts and negative things, you cannot do well. The way to have a clear mind is to fill your head with positive things. That makes me look at everything differently. I am better now at looking for the best in people."

When she is tempted to slack off, to skip her after-work walk in New York City, she looks back ten years to a time when she could not walk. She remembers the crippling severity of her osteomalacia, and then she puts on her workout clothes. "It's my way of saying, Thank you, Jesus. I can walk."

## THE RHYTHM OF RELAXATION

When walkers repeat words of praise or personal power, they trigger physical and mental reactions that reverberate on many more levels than they realize while they are exercising. First, by blocking out distracting worries or stresses, they put problems aside for a few minutes and experience a walk that provides a psychological break from the pressures of a demanding daily life. But the benefits go beyond the time of peace they enjoy during the actual walk.

By repeating a word, phrase, prayer, sound, or physical movement, we elicit what cardiologist Herbert Benson calls the "relaxation response." Benson, president of the Mind-Body Medical Institute of Harvard Medical School, identified the response in tests with students of transcendental meditation. His studies confirmed that meditative practices produced short-term calming effects and long-term health benefits that could be duplicated by the repetition of a sound, phrase, or movement pattern.[4] Benson found that meditators could achieve a relaxed state by simply repeating "one, one, one" with each breath, but he concluded later that people who select words with spiritual or personal significance are more likely to stick with the repetition and find enhanced value and satisfaction from the meditation.[5] In *Timeless Healing: The Power and Biology of Belief,* Benson suggests using words such as *love, peace,* and *ocean,* or phrases from religious sources that have personal meaning.[6]

Because both walking and repetition of meaningful words can evoke the benefits of relaxation, combining the two in an active, vigorous walking meditation strengthens both mental and physical benefits of the relaxation response. Walking meditation unites the energies of body and mind in an activity that brings greater mental clarity and long-term health benefits such as reduction of chronic pain and headaches, lessening of PMS symptoms, better sleep, and improved mental health.

Many teachers believe the benefits of affirmation extend even further. Shakti Gawain, author of *Creative Visualization,* says that if you are able to spend just ten minutes a day repeating effective positive affirmations you can reverse the damaging habits of negative self-talk and self-limiting beliefs. It isn't important whether the affirmations are spoken aloud, silently, written, sung, or chanted, she says.[7] The value comes with "affirming" or making a clear and positive statement about something you imagine.

If you still doubt the power of affirmations, consider the example of best-selling cartoonist Scott Adams. Creator of the phenomenally successful cartoon strip *Dilbert,* Adams majored in business economics and spent seventeen years in a corporate cubicle before he leaped off the white-collar ladder and onto the comic pages. He credits daily repetition of affirmations with his successful career change.[8] "I will become a syndicated cartoonist," he wrote fifteen times a day as he worked on developing a cartoon portfolio. When a syndicate purchased his strip, he revised the affirmation. "I will be the best cartoonist on the planet," he affirmed. Book buyers confirmed his success by pushing *The Dilbert Principle* and *Dogbert's Top Secret Management Handbook* onto the *New York Times* best-seller lists and bestowing on *Dilbert* a place in cartoon history beside *The Far Side* and *Calvin and Hobbes.*

When affirmations don't work, it may be that you've been wishy-washy about stating your goal. Nonchalance doesn't work with affirmations. Be realistic, but also be bold. State the affirmation in language that is positive and charged with feeling. Then be willing to do the work of repetition that gives the affirmation power. It also helps to give thanks each time you state or write an affirmation. Try creating affirmations that begin with gratitude. "I give thanks for health and fitness," for example. "I give thanks for the opportunities in my life." By giving thanks in advance, you create an attitude of appreciation and acceptance that encourages you to become aware of what you have rather than of what you lack.

Henry Ford is credited with a terse summary of the impact of our self-talk: "Whether you think you can, or think you can't, you're probably right."[9] The statement sounds like a contradiction, but it identifies an important truth: how you think and talk to yourself often determines what you achieve. When you integrate affirmation into your walking program, the repetition of your steps "re-affirms" and internalizes your words. Affirmation gives life to your imagination. It fuels your mental inventions.

# From Sole to Soul . . .

*Affirmative Action:* Affirmations are powerful tools for internal remodeling projects. They work by using words as the raw materials for mental makeovers. Repetition is the skill that installs them in your life.

Affirmations are statements that "affirm," or declare to be true, beliefs and outcomes that you want in your life. They offer clear evidence that the way you talk to yourself can change a lot of what you experience in life. When I wanted to remodel my self-image as a physical klutz, an affirmation helped me design the changes I wanted. We all have "modifications" we'd like to make in fitness level, exercise patterns, or self-image. A walking or fitness affirmation provides a do-it-yourself tool for taking action on remodeling projects that can update muscle and mind.

A good place to begin is with an affirmation that will help you establish a regular walking practice. Think about common complaints or concerns that interfere with your walking pleasure. What are the protests that come into your thoughts while you exercise? What excuses tempt you to skip your daily walk? How would you rather feel about exercise? Take a few minutes to think about how you would complete these phrases. Jot down the words that come to mind.

How I want to feel when I am walking is:

How I'd like my body to be when I am walking is:

62

How I'd like my mind to be when I am walking is:

The attitude that I'd like to have toward walking is:

Your responses will reveal words that have significance to you. For example, if you often find your steps dragging and your pace slowing because your legs feel tired, you might try an affirmation that states, *My legs are strong. I move with ease.*

If you get impatient or feel bored and want to cut walks shorter than your planned exercise time, you might create an affirmation that keeps you focused on the present: *I am here and I am happy. I am focused and full of joy.* If you feel tense and tight, consider words that affirm ease and relaxation. If you find it hard to settle into a comfortable, coordinated stride, try affirming that you are graceful, balanced, or smooth. If you just feel out of shape, choose words that affirm being fit, lean, healthy, or active.

State your affirmation in the present tense, as if it were already true. Create positive statements. Consider starting with the words *I am* or *I have.* Notice the enormous difference between: *I am strong* and *I am not weak.* Or *I have a strong, healthy body* as opposed to *I am going to have a strong, healthy body.* The first statements paint a bold image in the mind. Go for clear, positive words. If they feel outrageous and untrue at this time, try them anyway. Remember, you are creating an advertising slogan for yourself. No one else needs to hear it. You are selling to yourself now.

Play around with your affirmation for a few days. Sometimes the words will change slightly to create a clearer message. Keep experimenting until you are sure that you have an affirmation that truly clicks for you. To have impact in your life, it must accurately reflect your own visions, goals, or aspirations, not someone else's "shoulds."

If you can form a phrase that matches the rhythm of your steps, it will deepen the impact of the statement. As you chant your affirmation mentally, your words establish a rhythmic pattern that helps keep you moving. Some people like the melodic impact of affirmations that rhyme: *I am here and I am clear. I'm on a roll, moving forward with soul. I hit my stride, walking with pride.* Some people write affirmations in the form of lyrics to a song that they sing to themselves as they walk. If you want to try this, choose a song with a brisk beat that keeps your feet moving.

When you are satisfied with your affirmation, write it down where you will see it daily. Stick it up on the bathroom mirror for a month. Put it on a piece of paper and tuck it into a pocket of your walking jacket. Make it a part of daily life so that it becomes second nature to you. Then it can begin to work. Repeat your affirmation mentally as you walk.

Devote at least ten minutes to uninterrupted repetition of the affirmation during your walks or in the cooldown phase. Naturally your thoughts will wander from time to time, but you'll catch yourself eventually. Start over with the affirmation. Repetition helps train your beliefs and your mental patterns. Gradually, you will integrate the words, and the affirmation will slide into your awareness automatically, drawing you back to the goal you have chosen as your focus.

Remember that successful athletes train mentally as well as physically. Mental conditioning is a part of physical excellence. Those of us who aren't seeking to be elite athletes still can have bodies that perform with excellence in support of our daily lives. Affirmations are an integral part of the training program that will help us achieve this goal.

*Back Talk:* When you are ready to test the power of a walking or fitness affirmation, give yourself at least thirty minutes for this exercise, which provides opportunities to talk back to self-doubt. Choose a familiar route where you will be able to focus on your affirmation without traffic interruptions. Take five to ten minutes for a gentle warm-up and then stop for a couple of minutes to rotate your shoulders, hips, and ankles. This exercise asks that you push yourself, so it is important that you feel loose, warm, and ready for action before you begin.

A fifteen-minute interval workout forms the core of this workout. You will be alternating between intervals of fast, hard walking and segments of slower, recovery walking. As you move through it, you'll confront the internal voices that try to pull you off your fitness course. Your goal is to strengthen your body both mentally and physically by confronting resistance and moving beyond it.

Check your watch and fix in your mind a three-minute goal. Now, start walking at a pace that is faster than your usual walk. Push yourself. You may feel uncomfortable at this new speed, but remember it's only for three minutes. Your goal is to get your heart rate into the target rate zone that you identified in chapter 2. In terms of "perceived exertion," you want to feel that you are working "somewhat hard." It may be difficult to carry on a conversation during this segment. That's fine. Focus on maintaining the same speed for the entire interval.

At the end of three minutes, check your pulse. For cardiovascular benefit, you want to reach your target range. Slow your pace and continue walking for two minutes. Your heart rate should drop during this recovery phase. At the end of two minutes, check your watch and repeat the three-minute acceleration interval. If you don't have a watch, look ahead and pick out a lamppost, a tree, a mailbox, or another marker as your goal. Push yourself once again to a speed that is faster than usual for you. It should be vigorous enough that you need to focus your attention fully on your walking. Maintain that pace for three minutes.

You'll probably bump into the protesters before that three minutes is up. "This can't be good for you," they'll insist. "This is dumb. You look stupid. Walking should be enjoyable." This is your chance to talk back to the mental taunters that try to pull you off course.

"I am here and I am walking," I snap at the voices that nag me. "I am fit and fast and focused." Use your own affirmation as a tool to declare your intention to stay on course. Say it again and mean it. Over and over. The words keep you focused on your goal and block the noisy naysayers who complain about every change of pattern. Keep your attention on your words and your time goal. Use your affirmation to support your physical effort. At the end of three minutes, relax and walk slowly for two minutes. Then repeat the sequence a third time.

The interval workout looks like this:

*Interval A:* Three-minute speed walk at a brisk pace

*Interval B:* Two-minute recovery walk at reduced pace

*Interval A:* Three-minute speed walk

*Interval B:* Two-minute recovery walk

*Interval A:* Three-minute speed walk

*Interval B:* Two-minute recovery walk

During the exertion intervals, make an effort to push yourself beyond your comfort zone but not beyond your capacity. You are likely to feel the physical discomfort of hard work and unfamiliar effort, but you shouldn't experience pain. If you are not accustomed to listening to your body, increase your speed gradually. Checking your pulse at the end of each interval will help you interpret your body's responses. You'll also be able to monitor the changes in heart rate and recovery that occur with regular exercise.

Learning to use positive back talk to keep yourself moving in the direction and at the pace you want is a skill worth practicing on walks and in life. Try this exercise regularly. Including an interval workout in your walking schedule once a week will help you develop increased speed and focus.

# CHAPTER 4

~

## *Imagery for Walkers*
### Encounters with Tigers and Hawks

Residents of a rural neighborhood on the edge of town insisted that their peace of mind and personal safety were on the line when they launched a protest campaign against a neighbor. They complained to the county commission, the sheriff's office, and the local newspaper. The tiger in the backyard had to go. The tiger in question was a 225-pound Siberian female named Sheba who had been purchased as a pet when she was small. For eighteen months the owner had kept her in a chain-link cage behind the house. After she bit a visitor, neighbors raised an uproar. They wanted the tiger in a zoo, not in a backyard.

My editor put me on the story. To supplement the local paper's coverage of the conflict, he wanted a feature article about people who keep wild animals as domestic pets and about the laws that regulate their choices. When I arrived for an interview with the tiger's owner, we headed directly to the backyard. I stood a few feet away from the chain-link cage and watched in awe as the magnificent feline paced restlessly back and forth across the concrete floor of her enclosure. The constant motion intensified the sense of power confined in her sleek body. "Don't be nervous," the owner reassured me. "She paces all the time. She paces so much, she has sores on her feet, and she still won't stop."

The sight was painful to me. State regulations demanded a concrete-floor enclosure to prevent wild animals from digging free and endangering innocent people. But this cat's claws had been removed. Her cushioned paws were designed for earth and grass. The harsh concrete surface scraped the pads of her feet until they were scabbed and tender. Still, she stalked her cage, confined but not subdued.

I watched the cat from a respectful distance, mesmerized by the strength and determination in her stride. The image haunted me. After interviews with other wild-animal owners, I wrote an article and moved on to new assignments. But the tiger pursued me. In unexpected moments, I'd catch a glimpse of her in my mind's eye, patrolling her cage defiantly. What does she feel? What kind of energy compels her to pace a surface that produces constant pain? At some level, her restlessness seemed to connect with something restrained inside me—something powerful, stubborn, graceful,

69

defiant. Looking back, I recognize it now as my own physical strength, a part of me that was confined for long years within a cage of "appropriate" behavior: Don't get your clothes dirty. Don't jump on the bed. Stop squirming. Keep your voice down.

By the time I encountered the tiger, my sense of physical freedom had expanded. I had discovered the exhilaration of mountain hikes. I walked for exercise two or three days a week. One morning as I neared the end of my walk, feeling rushed and impatient to complete this task and get on with a busy day, the tiger flashed into my mind. Instead of seeing her confined in a cage, I imagined her beside me, walking on my neighbors' lawns as I matched her pace on the sidewalk. My stomach tightened with wariness. I felt cautious but fascinated. Given this freedom, would she race away? Would she turn on me in anger?

Soon my mind bounced off in other directions. The tiger slipped from my thoughts. A few days later, she showed up again as I walked. This time I smiled at her arrival. I picked up my pace and moved into step beside her, absorbing her power and energy. Even the imaginary presence of this splendid beast seemed to boost my adrenaline. Before long, my mind veered off into a tangle of details about the day ahead. When I looked up, I caught a glimpse of the tiger at the corner, twitching her tail in the impatient manner of cats.

"Come on, come on," she seemed to prod. "Let's go. Let's move. Let's race." The image delighted me. Given her freedom, she had not abandoned me, nor had she lost her strong willfulness. She walks with me now like an old friend, appearing in city parks or on mountain trails to keep me company. Sometimes I call her. Sometimes she surprises me and bumps me out of reveries. I feel her strong body brush against my thigh and instantly my own step changes. "Walk like a tiger," I remind myself. My shoulders lift. My chest opens to draw in a deep breath. My pace assumes a smooth elegance. I see it clearly in my mind—my body moving with the grace and ease of a cat. On days when I'm frustrated with my workout and battling the urge to toss it in, the tiger blocks my path. She snaps her tail in disbelief. "How can you question this freedom?" she protests. "How can you even consider quitting, once you've felt the whole-body joy of vigorous movement?"

The imaginary tiger has emerged as a metaphor for my own physical energy. When I see myself as a tiger, my body feels stronger, my pace becomes smoother. My muscles relax and walking feels easier, more natural. The visual image of her has the power to invigorate my step. It reminds me to have gratitude for a strong, healthy body and for the freedom to move.

## MAKE AN IMPRESSION

Visual images—the imaginary pictures we create in our minds—have very real impact in our lives. The way we see ourselves in personal relationships, at work, at a Saturday night party, or in a gym determines our attitudes and actions. Do we see someone strong and competent? Weak and vulnerable? Temperamental? Resourceful? Helpless?

That depends on the situation. At coffee with the quick-witted journalists I worked beside for years, I often saw myself as stumbling and slow. In my view, my comfort with words reveals itself in deliberation, not in clever replies. But ask me about preparing to do an interview and a completely different image emerges. This one shows me as confident and competent, notebook in hand and ready to ask questions.

One of my athletic mentors, a woman who held national titles as a distance runner during her competitive years and who ran with the world's top athletes, confided to me that the weight room of our health club terrifies her. In spite of her athletic achievements and physical ability on a track, she sees herself as a misfit in a gym. In her mind's eye, her lean runner's body looks out of place beside the sculpted muscles of weight-room regulars. She rushes through strength workouts with eyes down, avoiding connection with the people around her.

Fortunately, we have the ability to change many of the pictures we haul around in mental scrapbooks. Just as positive words have the power to reverse negative self-talk, visualization can reframe a warped self-portrait. Mental pictures are visual affirmations. They are powerful self-concepts interpreted in images or impressions rather than in words. Like affirmations, they have the power to shape the way we see ourselves in the world. Don't dismiss visualization as mental fluff or self-deception. Visualization doesn't simply cover up reality with rose-colored glasses. Like affirmations, it provides a tool with which we can redraw our view of the world. As with any tool, you have to *use* it to benefit from

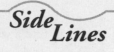

## A PICTURE OF SUCCESS

The gold stars that glittered at the top of school assignments or on the pages of a piano lesson book blazed a powerful image on my young mind. They symbolized achievement and approval. They sprinkled early lessons in life with an intoxicating glimpse of stardom that sent me off in search of more.

As an adult, I'm still motivated by stars. Gold stars, red stars, blue and yellow. I've branched out to embrace a rainbow of approval in the stickers I splash across my daily calendar when I achieve a personal goal. Visual evidence strokes my pride. That image of success at the top of the page sends me forward with renewed commitment and a glow of satisfaction.

As a source of motivation, almost nothing beats a record that gives you a visual image of your accomplishments. Useful tracking systems can be as simple as stars on your calendar every day that you walk or as sophisticated as a daily log. A record of walking distances, times, and speeds lets you monitor your progress as you build fitness. But more important, it can keep you on course when you find yourself distracted by other demands in your life.

Trainers say that people who take the time to make a few notes about workouts tend to remain committed to fitness goals. The self-discipline that you practice by recording your walks strengthens the discipline that keeps you going day after day in the pursuit of personal and fitness goals.

You don't need an elaborate record system or even a special notebook to create a method of visual motivation. If you already use a personal calendar, find a way to include walking details in your daily notations. Or simply copy pages from an ordinary calendar and keep one month at a time in a convenient spot where you will see it. Somewhere on the calendar, jot down your action goals for the month:

How many days do you intend to walk?

Or how many miles?

Perhaps your goal will be to make at least one walk each week a time to experiment, when you will try one of the exercises suggested at the end of each chapter in this book.

Each time you keep your goal, make a note of it on the calendar. Maybe you want to give yourself a star. If you'd like to enlarge your picture of success, begin to sketch in some more details:

Jot down the route you walked and how long it took.

Make a note of the distance if you know it.

Add a detail about the weather or your mood.

Did the workout seem easy or hard today?

Were you fast or slow? Did you maintain an aerobic pace?

If you love visual stimulation, use colored pens to record mileage, time, or mood. Get creative with stickers. I once found stickers shaped like running shoes, which I used to highlight personal bests or significant events. Be playful. Let your imagination kick up its heels as you create a visual system to support your fitness goals.

At the end of the week, add up the number of minutes you walked. Or total up the miles you covered. You may watch both increase as you maintain a commitment to fitness. Perhaps you'll find a pattern that tells you what time of day you walk best and most efficiently. You'll also see improvements in speed and aerobic ability as your training advances.

You may learn to spot slowdowns that offer warning signs. Perhaps your body needs a day of rest. Maybe you need to drink more water. Keeping notes will help you learn to interpret physical indicators more accurately.

Each month, total up the number of days you walked. Compute the miles if you have them. How well did you do in meeting the action goals you set? How about giving yourself a special pat on the back if you've achieved a goal this month? A pair of new walking socks would be great. Or that book a friend raved about. Then write the reward on your log as evidence of your success.

Do you want to revise the goals or make changes in your exercise schedule next month? Reviewing the record each month helps you renew your commitment to body-mind fitness. After you've reviewed your walking log at the end of the month, stick the page in a drawer so you can look back at it as a reference when you want evidence of your commitment and your progress.

it. With deliberate focus and repetition, you can gain control over the automatic responses with which your mind has grown comfortable.

Mental imagery changes our reality because it transmits information to muscles and brain cells and carves new pathways for messages about physical movement and self-image. Just watching athletes on television or at community events can improve your own physical skills if you get up and imitate what you've seen, says research psychologist Steven Ungerleider. A powerful connection exists between seeing and doing, he says. Weekend skiers demonstrate improved skills after watching televised coverage of Olympic downhill competition. Recreational tennis players perform better after viewing a championship match. When we mentally record movements we'd like to copy, we trigger actual changes in muscle memory, he reports in *Mental Training for Peak Performance.*[1]

As you incorporate visualization into your walks, you will bolster athletic performance and strengthen an image of yourself as a fit and active person. Keep your eyes open for walkers or athletes who move in a manner you'd like to imitate, and snap a mental picture for inspiration. Then let your imagination play with the image.

When I decided to participate in a sport that most of the world considers funny-looking, friends and family were mystified. They know me as a person who hates to look foolish. "Racewalking?" they'd ask incredulously. "Isn't that where you do weird stuff with your hips?" For them, the word produced a mental picture of a stiff-legged racewalker strutting awkwardly across a movie screen. A buffoon. But I had a different image. A couple of years before, I had watched a tall, lean woman move around a track with a speed and poise that intrigued me. I thought that I had never seen such athletic elegance in an adult. Later, when I decided to pick up my own walking pace and adopt racewalking form, it was her image I carried in my mind. If acquaintances teased me with joking imitations, I shrugged their jests aside. "My fantasy is that I look elegant," I'd laugh. "Let me have my illusions." What I called "fantasy" was simply another word for the strong, positive visual image that shaped my attitude toward racewalking.

Even now, on days when my body feels stiff and awkward and my feet land heavily on the ground, I pull out my well-worn mental picture and imagine her moving gracefully ahead of me. I fix my eyes on the French braid that ladders down the back of her head and let my body find the rhythm of her steps. My legs get longer, my torso taller. Instead of seeing myself as sluggish and stiff, I feel my energy rise as my muscles adopt a graceful, easy pattern of movement.

Whether we call them fantasies, daydreams, or active imagination, we all have experienced visualization. Often it emerges without conscious thought. Sometimes those unconscious visualizations discourage us from pursuing fitness goals or put a damper on our enthusiasm. We see pictures of past embarrassments. We remember struggling to please a coach or a parent. Old impressions linger in the mind to block the sense of adventure and the willingness we once had for physical exercise. Sometimes we let comparisons limit our view. We shudder at a mental image of ourselves in workout clothes. We're afraid of lagging behind on a walk with friends. It's easy to let those images inflate until they block the path to our dreams and goals. Studies of overweight people clearly indicate that poor self-image, rather than lack of desire, inhibits participation in fitness activities.[2] By consciously deciding to replace limiting images with pictures that expand our options, we open our minds and our lives to new achievements.

Imagine what would happen to successful athletes if they clung tenaciously to every mistake. Even the most talented performers would quickly become has-beens if they couldn't redirect their focus after disappointments. Visualization allows them to take responsibility. It lets them decide what pictures will control their performances. If you watch championship competitions, you see the process at work. In the moment of silent concentration that signals final preparation, many athletes pause for a mental practice run. They focus on an image of themselves moving in perfect form and completing their event successfully. Whether that pause comes at the edge of a high-dive board or in the starting gate of a downhill ski course, it unites the mental and physical training an athlete has done in preparation for competition.

The same tool is available to all of us. Fitness walkers may not need such intense preparation for an exercise outing, but we can certainly energize and motivate ourselves before a walk by choosing positive mental images. With selective imagery, we control the barrage of pictures that flash helter-skelter through our minds and trip up good intentions.

## GET THE PICTURE

Advertising demonstrates the effectiveness of imagery in shaping our opinions and actions. We choose our clothing, our vacation spots, even our hair color on the basis of pictures and slogans that have been pressed into memory with vivid words and scenes. Repetition locks them in place. Advertisers hope we'll accept unconsciously the images they create, and often we do. But when we become *aware* of the mental pictures that guide our behaviors, we gain the power to choose.

Kay Porter, a therapist and runner who teaches mental skills for athletic and personal clarity, suggests that the place to start in creating a strong, active image is sitting down. Close your eyes and imagine that you are at the seashore or a favorite lake. What do you notice first? Do you see waves rolling in? Boats on the horizon? Stretches of white sand? Do you hear the roar of the sea? Smell the crab pots? Feel the movement of a cool breeze? What you pay attention to first often determines which sense is dominant in your imagination. Include that sense when you create a mental image of fitness or healthy vigor. Then, if you give your vision lots of air time as you walk, like an aggressive advertising campaign, it will upgrade the quality of your outings, bringing increased energy and awareness. It can even boost a commitment to exercise. Remember that successful advertising usually involves more than pictures. Round out the scene with sounds and feelings and you'll have a vivid vision with the power of a well-made commercial.

When Porter, the highly visual coauthor of *The Mental Athlete*,[3] gears up for her own fitness workouts, she turns to mental imagery for motivation. She finds that simply thinking about the beautiful, natural settings where she often runs moves her into action. Flowering trees inspire her in springtime. Fall colors draw her outside in autumn. Images from nature remind her of the value she receives from exercise. They support her in keeping her commitment to fitness and health. "Nature motivates me to get outside. How I nourish my soul is from nature. I think about the earth and the sky and the wind and the rain and everything I see. When I walk or run, I am grateful a lot. Even on bad days, I am grateful for a lot," she says.

Imagery that inspires and encourages provides a powerful energizing force in a walking program. Instead of approaching every workout through the battering gauntlet of "shoulds" and "have-tos" that often accompany fitness resolutions, use mental images to remind you of your walking goals. Find a focus that connects your vision and your spirit, the way Porter's trees trigger her love of nature. Or the way my imaginary tiger reminds me how much I value freedom and physical movement. Nature is a loyal ally for those who seek connection, awareness, and a sense of wonder in their lives.

A few years ago, my husband and I participated in a community walkathon and joined a pack of walkers marching through city streets. At first, the crowd's enthusiasm filled us with energy. Then, as the starting-line exhilaration faded, we settled into the monotony of a long walk. We felt our spirits slump. Suddenly my husband pointed toward the sky. "Ah," he announced. "Red hawk soars on the wind." The image was familiar. In the agricultural valley where we live, highway travel provides spectacular viewings of these predatory birds. At the edge of the road, hawks lift silently from fence posts and soar above the stubble of mowed crops in search of prey. Now, without a bird in the sky, we could see the power of that ascent and the ease and control of the bird's movement. We felt it move through our own muscles and lift our bodies effortlessly. I hadn't known that my husband used animal imagery to revitalize his spirits and his pace. Perhaps he didn't know it either. The image appeared and he grabbed it mentally, choosing to hold it for a few moments as an uplifting picture of movement and ease.

## BECOMING A VISIONARY

If visualization can halt the spread of cancer, make warts disappear, and speed the healing of wounds, as growing medical evidence suggests, doesn't it make sense that imagery is powerful enough to heal emotional wounds, as well? Many people grow up with an image of themselves as nonathletic and uncoordinated. Women, especially, share this view because so many of us were not encouraged to participate in community and school sports programs. But even outstanding athletes struggle with self-image. Athletes who achieve high school and collegiate recognition consider themselves failures when they can't maintain the same level of performance as they age. Others develop such a strong imperative for perfection that they see themselves as failures anytime they miss a cue. We all walk around with images in our minds every day. Some are pleasant, some unpleasant, some confused. When we actively practice mental visualization, we take responsibility for selecting imagery that will benefit us in a particular task.

My mental snapshot of the smooth, fluid walker I once watched on a track became a powerful vehicle for guiding me beyond a critical view of myself as awkward and nonathletic. By holding her image in my mind as I walked, I etched a new impression into my mental gallery. I was telling my body, *Hey, I like the way that person moves. I want to walk like that.* Researchers say such visualization can actually code new blueprints into our cells. Quite literally, I changed the way I moved and viewed myself.

Give your imagination lots of encouragement and creative freedom as you experiment with letting imagery reinforce your walking goals. In addition to imitating the movements of people you admire, tap into the energy of animals or the power of light as you sample the supportive force of visualization.

*Let the Sunshine In:* On a day when you feel yourself tiring and running out of steam, imagine a beam of brilliant sunlight pouring into the top of your head as you walk. See the light flowing through you in such abundance that it splashes out in puddles at your feet. Play in the light like a child—so much energy, so much radiance filling your life. Visualizing light is a simple technique that reminds us of the energy surrounding us at all times. Usually, we are so confined within the narrow concerns of our minds that we don't feel or acknowledge the connection we have with the physical and spiritual world around us and with sunlight, which fuels life on our planet. This simple image has a profound power to unify the energies of body, mind, and spirit.

*Create a Cord:* Effective visualizations can be as simple as pretending to have a cord attached to the top of your head, lifting you gently upright. Maybe you want cords from your shoulders to correct a drooping posture and ease the movement of your limbs. Feel the weight of your body change as cords on your head and shoulders gently support you. Meditation teacher Shunryu Suzuki emphasized the importance of posture to students at the San Francisco Zen Center. When the body slumps, the mind collapses, too, he warned.[4] His words hold equal wisdom for walkers. Let your chest cave in or your spine collapse and you'll soon feel tired and distracted. Mindfulness disappears. Mental cords can keep your posture tall. Feel your chest rise gracefully, free of the weight that burdens the body when you fragment your attention and splinter your energies.

*Martial a Power Source:* Whole-body walkers can borrow mental imagery tools from the martial arts. Moving meditation practices such as tai chi or aikido teach students to imagine that the source of power in the body rests low in the abdomen, just below the navel. By focusing on this center, students achieve physical balance and stability. Muscles are relaxed and able to respond smoothly rather than locked in rigid poses. This power center below the navel delivers the same stability to walkers. Imagine energy flowing from this center as you walk. See and feel the current pumping into your arms and legs with each step. Then let a beam of energy extend into a cord that enters your lower back and exits through the power core in the front. Hook that cord to a tree down the street ahead of you or to a light post a block away. Relax and allow the cord to pull you gently and steadily along your route, like a powerful bungee cord.

Years ago, I took my first ski lessons in a tiny ski area where chairlifts were unknown. Skiers reached the top of the slope on a simple poma lift, an overhead rope pulley that guided us up the hill along a tow track rutted with use. It was a delicate balancing act, requiring clear focus and relaxed muscles to slide safely over dips in the path. Sometimes I imagine that ski lift as I walk now, sensing the pressure of the pulley that eased me forward while I shifted my weight to maintain balance. The image connects me to a time when I was a beginner, struggling sometimes but open to new concepts and experiences. It is a good image to carry with me in the present.

Just as often, we carry into the present tattered images from the past that are no longer useful. These, too, can become powerful mental tools with a little retouching and updating. Steven Ungerleider knows firsthand the power of imagery to redraw old, automatic pictures and free us to move in new ways. Long before he began to explore the mental and physical training of top athletes as a research psychologist, he felt the pressure for peak performance in his own life. Athletic parents envisioned victories at Wimbledon as they groomed their son for tennis stardom. When they transmitted that vision through a rigorous training schedule, it produced nightmares for their child. He fled from tennis in a swirl of stress and anger. A sense of failure haunted him. Twenty-five years later, when his teenage daughter discovered tennis and begged her athletic dad to hit balls with her, old pictures blocked his swing. "Even as someone who has been an athlete most of my life, I struggle with self-image issues," he says. "I had to get rid of imagery from my past because I really wanted to enjoy playing with my daughter."

When we intentionally use mental skills to alter the way we think or move, we stop the automatic fast-forward action that occurs in our heads most of the time. By consciously focusing attention and awareness in one place, we move toward meditation and into the clear, still moment of the present. It's like the scan button on the radio in my kitchen. Hit the button and the signal picks up a station for a few seconds to let me sample the broadcast, before it races ahead automatically to the next strong signal it can find. Unless I actively stop the scan, this stop-start action continues endlessly—just like the signals in my head. Mental imagery stops the scan and puts the station on hold for a time. It makes an active choice about the information I want to receive.

Meditation teacher Eknath Easwaran offers a colorful picture to illustrate the way the mind leaps from one thing to the next, distracting us from our purpose.[5] In his native India, Easwaran says, villages often celebrated holy days with processions of musicians and elephants. Imagine an elephant weaving through the crowds, its restless trunk snatching fruit from stands along the narrow streets. Here a mango. There a papaya. Now a nice banana. In addition to the problem of stolen fruit, for which a merchant wanted payment, the procession would bump along at a fitful pace. To keep the procession headed toward its destination, the elephant trainer would give the animal a distraction. Having the elephant hold a stick or baton in its trunk handled the situation. With this task to carry out, the elephant moved dutifully along the route without being drawn to other temptations. The mind, Easwaran says, is a similar animal. It needs a stick to hold when you want to keep your focus clear and narrow. Give it a word, a vision, a prayer—the sticks of meditators.

# From Sole to Soul . . .

*The Tao of Walking:* In recent years, the word *tao* has been absorbed into English usage as a New Age synonym for the core truth or spiritual essence of everything from sex to money. A Chinese word, *tao* means "the way." Usually it implies the way of nature—a route or method that works in harmony with the energy of the earth and of all life. Many martial arts regard walking as the natural way for humans to practice balance, strength, and concentration.

This exercise introduces walking variations on ancient practices that teach alignment of mind and motion through exercise and calisthenic routines. Allow thirty minutes. You'll want a flat route where you can walk a straight line for five to ten minutes without the interruption of crosswalks or traffic lights. Allow yourself a few minutes of warm-up to settle into your body and loosen muscles and joints before you begin.

Focus your attention on the area just below your navel, the body's center of energy and stability in the martial arts. As you begin to walk, notice your posture; then turn your attention back to the body's center. Feel your weight become solidly balanced in this area. Let your neck and shoulders relax. Arms swing easily and legs move effortlessly beneath you.

Now imagine that the weight of your body is resting on a golden monorail track that passes through the energy center in your pelvis. Let yourself glide smoothly forward on the flow of the current. Ride the rail as far as you can, noticing that your legs lift easily. Your body actually feels lighter as you let the track carry you along. Perhaps you feel the speed picking up as you accelerate with the current of the monorail. Breathe deeply. See if you can keep your focus and pace steady for five to ten minutes of walking.

Now take a break for thirty seconds of vigorous movement. Run rapidly in place, pumping your arms energetically to work the entire body and increase circulation. Or stand with feet apart and swing your arms around your body, one in front and the other in back so that you twist at the waist. Whip the arms around with unrestrained, dynamic energy, moving as fast as you comfortably can. You won't look any more unusual than people who jog at intersections while waiting for streetlights to change.

Pause for a moment to regain stability. Notice the energy surging through your body. Take a deep breath. Then return your focus to the monorail track and set off on another five- to ten-minute segment of centered, balanced walking. Some forms of moving meditation, such as Qi Gong, use rapid, dynamic activity to raise energy and increase concentration. Students alternate periods of vigorous jumping and dancing with sitting or walking meditation. You can experiment with this concept by inserting short bursts of high-energy movement into your walks as a way to revive energy and restore focus.

*Totem Energy:* In most parts of the world, your choices are fairly limited when you decide to select a pet. If you want an animal that can walk with you, dogs pretty much dominate the field. But when it comes to selecting a symbolic, or totem, animal to accompany your steps and inspire your journeys, an entire zoo opens for your inspection.

How will you know where to begin in selecting an animal companion to invite on your walks? Pretend that you are a child. Do you remember when your imagination soared with the delights of make-believe? When you could become anyone you wanted and perform incredible feats? Dust off those skills for this exercise. The power hasn't left you, as you'll discover when you complete this simple phrase:

"If I were an animal, I would be a . . ."

What came to your mind? Just say it. Fast. No need for analysis or deep contemplation. "If I were an animal, I would be a . . ." What's there? A horse, a deer, an eagle, a chipmunk, an elk? No matter. This animal wants to walk with you. Stop right now and consider the animal that came to you at the first flash of your imagination. Just observe without judgment. What do you notice about it that delights you? Intrigues you? Inspires you? What words do you use to describe how it moves? Just say them. Don't think. Don't struggle. Your imagination can handle this task. What can you learn from walking with this animal? Quickly. You know the answers. Sometimes your responses will surprise you. It's OK to laugh as you do this exercise. Be a child. Free your caged imagination.

Then invite this animal to accompany you on your next exercise outing. As you walk, imagine it moving beside you, or leading you, the way my tiger sometimes does. Find something in the animal's walk or in its use of energy that you can imitate with your own body and spirit. How does it feel to be a zebra or a wolf? What can you learn from this companion that can assist you in your walking practice? Or in your life?

I suggest that you repeat this experiment several times. Invite a variety of animals along on walks before you adopt a totem animal. A totem animal has special significance. In many cultures it is believed that there is a natural connection or affinity between that animal and the person to whom it appears. Sometimes we reveal that affinity in our domestic pets. We identify ourselves as "a cat person" or "a dog person," as if those labels explained something significant about us. And they do. If you already feel drawn to a particular animal, it may be a subconscious link between you and the animal that is your kindred spirit in the natural world. Encourage that relationship. Learn from it and enjoy the adventure as you allow its energy to transform your gait and your spirit. Use it to deepen awareness of your connection with all nature.

## CHAPTER 5

~

# *Breathwork for Walkers*
## IN-TWO-THREE, OUT-TWO-THREE

On Saturday mornings, Donna and I used to meet at the bike path beside the river for walks that took us farther and faster than the workouts we squeezed into weekdays. Walking together made it easier to increase distance and duration once a week. Very quickly, the mornings developed a pattern. The first half mile was slow and easy. We caught up on events of the past week while our bodies adjusted to a warm-up pace.

When we reached the water fountain, we'd pause for a few minutes of easy stretching to flex hamstrings, thighs, and shins. Nothing vigorous, just gentle bends and a few rotations at the shoulders, waist, and ankles to loosen joints and muscles. We'd blow our noses, get a drink of water, and prepare to pick up momentum on the next leg of the walk.

The path from the fountain to the footbridge followed a smooth, level course along the riverbank. It was a good section for focusing attention on walking form and for pushing ourselves with the increased effort that would carry us into an aerobic workout zone. But sometimes an unfinished conversation followed us down the path. Soon we'd be talking as fast as we walked, moving on automatic along the familiar route. Conversation provided a pleasant distraction. We didn't think much about it when one or the other of us pulled to a stop with a moan. "Oh," we'd gasp apologetically. "Side ache. Got to slow down for a minute."

For months we found ourselves stumbling over cramped muscles in the course of our Saturday walks. We'd pause to stretch and inhale a few deep, relaxing breaths. We were slow to identify the pattern. Side aches, we eventually determined, occurred most often when we increased exertion without decreasing conversation. Reluctantly, we concluded that talking interfered with the deep rhythmic breathing that enables the body to perform efficiently, especially when increased demands are being made.

"Without proper breathing, even the best-conditioned athletes can get easily winded and fatigued and perform poorly," confirms sport psychologist Steven Ungerleider.[1]

An accomplished athlete himself, Ungerleider considers well-developed breathing skills the secret of athletic excellence. He's not alone in his appreciation. Conscious breathing is a tool of peak performers everywhere, a resource valued by athletes, meditators, entertainers, therapists, healers, and all who seek the clarity to pursue a vision.

By the time Donna and I teamed up to teach walking classes for the city parks department, we were familiar with the warning signs of unconscious breathing. "I can't keep this up," a student would gasp midway through a class workout. One of us would fall into step beside the discouraged walker. We'd hear the rapid inhalations that pump air in and out of the throat without getting much into the lungs. "Slow your breath," we'd suggest. "In-two-three, Out-two-three, In-two-three, Out-two-three, Breathing-in-to-the-bel-ly." The words set a cadence that brought miraculous changes. When students followed the rhythm of our words, they discovered a way to control the pace and depth of their breathing. Faces relaxed. Shoulders dropped. They tapped into a channel of energy that reached deep into the body instead of ending in gasps at the neck.

Steady deep breathing calms the mind and relaxes muscles. It offers an antidote to automatic responses that distract and disable us. Regulated breathing triggers a built-in system of control and connection. But you know that already. You've probably even prescribed it. "Relax," you advise a fretful friend. "Take a deep breath. You'll be fine." Then you watch a transformation take place. For a moment, disquieting fears disappear. Breath spreads through the body like a soothing breeze.

Several languages acknowledge the essential connection between breath and spirit or life by using the same word for both. In Latin, the word *spiritus* means both breath and spirit. The Sanskrit language speaks of *prana,* the life force carried in the breath. English places spirit at the essential core of life in the words *inspire* and *expire.* Still, we often forget that breath contains the miracle of life. We take the body's ability to breathe for granted and get caught short in situations where physical or emotional stress takes our breath away. In times of fear or anger or physical effort, breathing patterns become shallow. We literally cut ourselves off from what we need most. We suffer, not from a lack of information, but rather from a lack of practice.

The power of deep rhythmic breathing to enhance physical, mental, and spiritual well-being forms the foundation of many ancient spiritual and healing practices. In contemporary Western cultures, breath has gained new respect as medical research traces the source of many diseases to the stresses of modern life. Traditional techniques of relaxation and meditation use the breath as a focusing device to still the mind and quiet the distracting chatter of a demanding world. If you are consciously following each breath in and out of the body, your thoughts can't be racing around the grocery store or making plans for Saturday's soccer game. But breathing is more than a form of mental discipline. Breath links the inner and outer worlds, unifying action and intention. It guides us across the communication gaps that develop when mind and body are separate. We are given this key to connection and renewal as a birthright. Learning to use it with skillful appreciation requires practice. By developing awareness of the breath, we become better listeners for the physical information we receive from our own bodies.

Saturday morning side aches introduced me to the power of breath and to the subtleties of body language. When I learned to interpret the cramping in my side as a reminder to pay attention to basic breathing, I found a key to information that I'd been translating incorrectly for years. Body language has much to offer, but until you know how to listen, it's very easy to get the message wrong. For instance, how often have you decided that a side ache or shortness of breath while exercising is proof that you are:

A. Out of shape

B. Getting old

C. Exercising too hard

D. All of the above?

Before you accept any of those conclusions, try an experiment. When you begin to feel fatigued and tense on a brisk walk, see if you can reduce the symptoms simply by changing your breathing. Focus on your breath, thinking "in" as you inhale and "out" as you exhale. Keep your breathing steady and pull the air deep into the lungs so that you feel your abdomen rise and fall. If you are exercising at an aerobic level, you will probably find it easiest to breathe through the mouth. Maintain a brisk pace while slowing the rhythm of your breathing. Counting steps may help you stay focused. Three or four steps for each in-and-out breath is usually comfortable. It doesn't matter if you have the same number of steps on the inhale as on the exhale. Eventually they will even out, but for now, it is only important to stay focused on breathing. Soon you'll hear distractions in your mind: *Oh, this is working. I'm breathing better now. I wonder what the weather forecast is for Saturday.* Just return your focus to the breath. Continue to count your steps, pulling your awareness back each time it wanders.

Perhaps you'll find that the exhaustion you were feeling disappears. It's tremendously freeing to discover that fatigue arises sometimes from the lungs, not from the legs. Gasps for air signal the body's need for oxygen and for focused, rhythmic breathing. Consider those gasps respiratory hunger pangs and treat them with a fresh supply of nourishing air.

## INVEST IN BREATHING SPACE

Like affirmation and visualization, awareness of the breath is a meditation technique with the power to expand fitness walks into workouts for body, mind, and spirit. The unique contribution of breathing meditation is that it deepens the union of body and mind by using a biological process as the focus of attention. The breath links body and mind, leading to greater awareness of the physical sensations that arise during exercise.

# Side Lines

## On the Home Stretch

Stretching is a practice of gentleness in which we gradually increase our range and comfort zones. It eases the body's transition from action to rest. It improves balance, coordination, and circulation. It helps prevent muscle soreness after exercise. Still, we often find time stretched so thin that we cut workouts short and dash to the shower without stretching muscles. Be patient with yourself, but be firm and consistent as you develop mental and physical balance by making stretching a regular part of your fitness program.

The most thorough stretching should be done at the conclusion of an aerobic workout when muscles are warm. Cool down with five minutes of easy walking to let the body recover from an aerobic effort. Then fine-tune your mind and muscles by relaxing the major muscle groups that have been contracted during exercise. Move into each stretch slowly and hold the position without bouncing or putting pressure on the joints. Make your breathing deep and steady as you stretch and you will increase the relaxation of the muscles.

Allow your mind to focus on each set of muscles as you bring awareness to the stretch. Express your gratitude for a strong body as you exhale into each position. Acknowledge the healthy choices you are making.

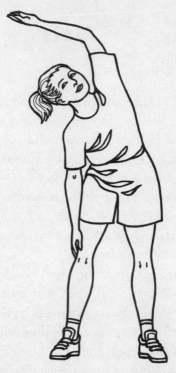

## SIDE STRETCH

Stand with knees apart and slightly bent. Smoothly raise one arm over your head. Relax the other arm and let it hang at your side. Exhale and bend slowly toward the arm that is hanging. Reach tall with the overhead arm so that you feel a stretch that extends from fingertips to hip. Hold the position without bouncing for a count of twenty. Repeat on the opposite side. To deepen the stretch into the hip, cross the right leg over the left, as if you are waiting for the bathroom. Keep the weight on both feet. Raise the right arm overhead and bend to the left. You should be able to feel the stretch in the hip joint. Repeat on the other side.

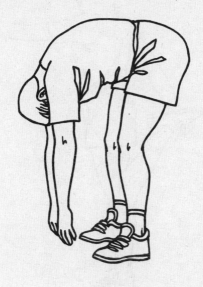

## HAMSTRING STRETCH

Walkers ask a lot of the hamstrings, the muscles that extend from the buttocks to the knee at the back of the thigh. Help them relax after a workout with a gentle forward bend, like a modified toe touch. Stand with feet about one foot apart and knees slightly bent. Lean forward slowly from the waist, letting your hands and head hang limp in front of you. Just let the body drape over without straining to touch the toes. Relax and breathe for a count of twenty; then slowly raise the body, rolling up one vertebra at a time. Repeat two times.

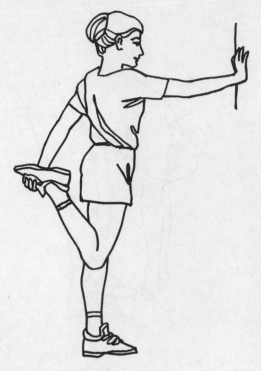

## THIGH STRETCH

Relax the hardworking quadriceps muscles of the thigh with a stretch you've seen lots of times. Place one hand on a tree or wall for balance and stand on the opposite foot, knee bent slightly so that you do not lock the joint. Lift the other foot behind you, bending it at the knee. Reach around your back with the free arm. Grab the toes and gently lift the foot toward the buttocks. Keep your knees together as you do this stretch. If you do not feel a comfortable stretch in the upper thigh, tilt the base of the pelvis forward gently, still keeping the knees together. Hold for a count of twenty and switch sides.

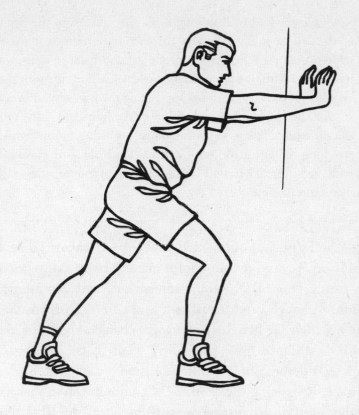

## CALF STRETCH

Stand about three feet from a wall or tree with both feet facing straight ahead. Lean toward the wall and place your hands on it at shoulder height. Step forward with one leg, bending the forward knee and keeping the toe straight ahead. Straighten the back leg, imagining that you are extending it down into the ground through the heel. You should feel a gentle stretch along the back of the straight leg. Exhale as you increase the stretch. Hold for a count of twenty and switch legs.

*Ankle Circles:* Brisk walking flexes the muscles in the front of the calf that lift the toes. To relax and strengthen these seldom-used muscles, stand on one leg and balance against a tree or wall with one hand. Make slow, deliberate circles in the air with the foot of the raised leg. Rotate the foot several times in each direction to release tension in the joint and shin. You can do more of these ankle rotations in waiting rooms, while watching TV, at the movies—whenever you are sitting around with free time. They will strengthen important muscles and increase walking ease.

Until I began pushing myself as a speed walker, I'd never fully experienced the unity of mind and body that relies on a steady flow of sensation, adjustment, and communication. Although I didn't realize it at the time, I'd spent most of my adult life like the James Joyce character who "lived at a little distance from his body."[2] Half of the messages I picked up were garbled in transmission—vague and unclear to me. Reopening the channels of communication that had fallen into disuse during years of living in my head took a lot of walking. The connection began to clear after I screwed up my courage and joined a handful of racewalkers for workouts with a coach. Physical fitness was only one component of the training program I stepped into at the track. These workouts demanded a singleness of focus I had never experienced before. Competition pushed my steps to a pace that demanded the full participation of both mind and muscle.

"Breathe!" my coach would shout from the sidelines during workouts. "Breathe!" he commanded again and again.

"Keep breathing. Dig down deep. Don't slow down." Sometimes the words provoked my anger. I didn't want to dig deep; I wanted to sit down. This kind of physical control was new to me. I didn't know how to keep my focus steady when my legs felt wobbly. Workouts became a battle between defiance and discipline.

Mind-body researcher Joan Borysenko maintains that all meditation incites the same conflict. "Meditation is a form of mental martial arts," she says. Eventually, we become skillful enough to move gracefully aside and not engage in the battle. "It's not that the mind stops attacking, but that we learn to take a different stance toward the attack."[3] For me, that change of stance emerged as my mind assumed the role of inner-coach. With practice and persistence, it learned to subdue the internal critic who interprets any sign of weakness as failure: *You'll never be able to do this. Why bother? Give it up.* Instead of fighting the protests that tumble through the mind on the heels of boredom or fatigue, my inner coach began to interpret them as distress signals from a mind that had drifted off course. *Breathe,* I'd remind myself. Fresh air awoke me to the moment, made me feel focused and fully conscious. *Breathe,* I'd repeat. *In and out. Here and now. I am here and I am breathing.* Breath opens a pathway for "digging down deep" and uncovering hidden reserves.

Begin teaching yourself to hear the voice of a supportive inner coach urging you to "breathe" whenever you feel fatigued. That voice will return your attention to the goal of walking with awareness. Allow the coach to subdue the critic who will leap up to berate you for letting your mind wander. Instead of focusing on shortcomings, thank the coach for waking you. Then focus on breathing in and out. When you learn to let oxygen restore cells and focus, you hold the key to living in the present, connected with your body.

Now, let the breath open another path of awareness. With each breath, follow the flow of air through your body for a posture scan. Very often, shortness of breath signals a slumping torso. Start at the top of your head and realign posture with each inhalation. Is your spine straight and tall? Chin tucked slightly? Shoulders relaxed? Think about exhaling tension from the upper back. Are your arms swinging freely at your sides? Does each foot hit the ground with balance and roll smoothly through to the toe? Maybe you want to shrug the shoulders a couple of times. Flex the fingers to loosen wrists and arms. Then return your focus to the breath and simply follow it in and out.

Breathing in gives life; breathing out brings cleansing, releasing impurities from the cells. The average person repeats the cycle twenty thousand times a day and rarely gives it a thought.[4] As a result, few of us appreciate this source of alertness, vitality, and health until we run short of it. Conscious breathing energizes the body, calms the emotions, and sharpens the mind. Researchers say it also slows the loss of vital lung capacity that often accompanies aging. Aerobic activity boosts the body's need for oxygen enormously and stimulates deeper breathing. As you breathe in fresh oxygen, you bring vital resources to the cells of the body and preserve the elasticity of lung tissue. You protect your capacity to live life fully. At the same time, production of carbon dioxide mounts as cells flush out waste products. Full exhalation releases spent resources that linger in the base of the lungs. Quite literally, it gives the body more room to breathe.

The symbolism of the breath establishes the flow of give and take as the essence of life. It guides us into a fundamental rhythm of release and renewal, of receiving and letting go. When you walk aerobically, think about breathing out tired thoughts, old frustrations, worn-out patterns along with the old air. Writer Shakti Gawain suggests that each exhalation provides an opportunity to "release an old way of life that no longer works for you." Every time you let go of old limits, you make space for something new, she says. When you inhale, imagine that "you are breathing in life energy, the life force of the universe."[5]

The coupling of rhythmic movement with deep breathing intensifies the meditative goal to "be here now." When you pay attention to each breath, awareness is fixed right here, right now. Conscious breathing supplies a key that locks out fears about the future: *I'm only half done; I'll never finish at this pace.* It blocks the passage to regrets about the past: *I started too fast. I stayed up too late last night.* Each breath renews a whole-body commitment to the present, to being fully alive and aware of the moment.

When walking becomes a vigorous, focused meditation, it closes the distance we often imagine between body and brain. It brings us closer to the union suggested by Zen master Shunryu Suzuki. Those who maintain that body and mind are the same thing are wrong, he says. Those who believe they are two separate things are also wrong. Those who see body and mind as two sides of the same coin move closer to the truth—two faces of a single unit.[6]

The coin image provides a reminder that I carry with me as I walk. In order to obtain the spiritual and physical wholeness I seek, I have to invest the whole coin. Just as I can't feed a parking meter with one side of a quarter, I can't satisfy my spirit with half of the body-mind. Spirited walking requires the whole coin. It asks for an effort that reaches beyond what's easy and automatic. It raises challenges that bring physical and mental resources together. With that union, we purchase a sense of wholeness that often eludes us.

Modern conveniences isolate us from the natural rhythms of the earth and our own bodies. As a result, we feel uncomfortable, unfamiliar, and maybe even a little embarrassed by the physical side of who we are. Breath carries us back into awareness of the body and into contact with the energy that flows constantly from inner to outer and back again. Conscious breathing reconnects us with the language of the body. It provides a pathway to information that supports and strengthens both sides of the whole-body coin.

## LISTEN TO YOUR BODY TALK

Sometimes just getting out of bed in the morning sets off a burst of body talk strong enough to change the course of your day. *My knee feels stiff—I'd better take it easy,* you tell yourself as you decide to skip your morning walk. *My calf muscle is sore—better give it some rest.* So you sit out a day or maybe two, torn between fear of an injury and guilt about failing to keep your exercise commitment. Just when you thought you'd found a way to increase the intensity and frequency of exercise, good intentions fall victim to the clamor of protesting muscles.

Without the expertise of a coach or personal trainer, how do you know when to pull back on an exercise program and when to keep pushing yourself? "Listen to your body," fitness advisers say. Unfortunately, people who have not exercised consistently and intensely often find that advice bewildering. "The inexperienced exerciser doesn't know how to interpret pain, and they get frightened when something hurts," says Stephanie Harris, a neurologist who is also a certified aerobics instructor and educator. "From my personal experience, if I listened only to my body and quit whenever anything was sore, I'd be inactive all the time."[7]

Effective listening requires both body and mind. People who exercise regularly learn the nuances of body language. They recognize the difference between stiffness and injury. Mastery begins with good warm-up skills. Ease into an aerobic workout with five to ten minutes of moderate walking. Use the warm-up to do a mental body scan: How are you feeling? Do you notice any twinges or tight muscles? "Warm-up is really important," Harris says. "The warm-up lets you get in tune with where you are physically and mentally." Even with a safe, low-impact activity like walking, you may feel some body stiffness when you exercise regularly. Warm-up allows the muscles to loosen gradually as you increase blood circulation through the body. A thorough walking warm-up should conclude with a few simple rotations of the arms, shoulders, waist, and ankles to increase flexibility. As you move through the rotations, keep your movements smooth and flowing. Check in with the muscles. If muscle tightness persists, revise your workout and exercise at a slower pace. As a rule of thumb, it takes about three weeks for the body to adjust to the demands of a new level of exercise.[8] People who rush to conclusions, abandoning an exercise program before their muscles adapt, never learn to understand body language. They are people who launch fitness programs and then drop out after two or three classes. Often they give sore muscles full authority for a decision that needs to be shared by the brain. "Listening to your body may mean taking a day off if you are really sore, but not stopping completely," Harris says.

Fluency comes with practice. Experienced exercisers realize that there are ups and downs in their lives and in their workouts, Harris says. They know that most of the time if they stick with a workout, they'll feel better at the end. This knowledge carries them through the initial stiffness that often accompanies warm-up. It enables them to evaluate their physical condition more accurately. People who bolt with the discomfort that may accompany the start-up phase of a new exercise program limit themselves to a life of repetition within a narrow range of motion. But even new exercisers can usually recognize the difference between tight muscles and the sharp pain of injury. Until muscles become accustomed to a new exercise program, you can expect some stiffness. If pain is persistent or sharp and it does not diminish with ten or fifteen minutes of easy warm-up, you may want to exercise at a lighter level that does not stress the muscles but allows you to maintain an exercise habit. If you have serious concerns about your physical ability to continue an exercise program, consult your physician or check with an exercise physiologist or knowledgeable fitness trainer at a health club.

Stretching helps protect the body against injury and significantly expands the opportunity to listen and learn from the body. Stretching creates flexibility. It enables the body to respond to challenges with balance and grace. It safeguards against rigidity. It keeps the body agile and limber. It reaffirms the exquisite union of body and mind. If body and mind are two sides of the same coin, true balance requires a suppleness that is both mental and physical.

Unfortunately, even people who achieve peak aerobic fitness often fail to recognize the contribution that stretching makes to whole-body fitness. It is the first casualty of busy schedules and a frequent victim of impatience. The safest and most extensive stretching should be done at the end of a workout, when muscles are warm. The harder you exercise, the more you need to stretch. Stretching releases tension in muscles that have been contracted during an activity. It's like taking a vacation or kicking back on the weekend after an intense workweek. You restore balance to the muscles and wellness to the body by relaxing systems that have been stressed. A careful balance of exertion and relaxation contributes to total well-being.

Slow, focused stretching fuses the mindfulness of meditation with the physical relaxation of deep breathing. It restores a sense of balance in the mind and body. A few essential stretches for walkers are suggested in this chapter.

When you want to increase your fluency in this area of body awareness, enroll in a yoga class or check out video and audio tapes that can guide you through a full-body stretch at the end of a vigorous walk. Stretching adds value that is both physical and spiritual.

As a physician, mother of preteen children, wife, and high-energy fitness enthusiast, Harris rarely slowed down long enough to stretch until she taught an aerobics class. There, medical wisdom took over. To her surprise, ten minutes of stretching at the end of workouts brought a sense of satisfaction that no other athletic pursuit provided. "At the end of a stretch period, there is this feeling of well-being," she says. "Stretching brings the cardiovascular workout to a conclusion. It's a sense of, 'Boy, this workout felt good.'"

## SPIRITED HAND-OUTS

When an acquaintance offered to teach me a new technique for meditative breathing, I accepted eagerly. In China, she said, she had learned to walk while breathing through her hands. My own breath patterns had never exceeded the confines of nose and mouth. The possibility of opening new channels of inhalation intrigued me.

We met on a patio outside her university office, and I watched as she stood in the sunlight, quieting her mind in preparation for the walk. Arms bent at the elbow, she turned the left hand down, facing the earth. She turned the right palm toward the sky. As she stepped forward, she swung the opposite arm forward in a normal walking gait and began a rhythmic breathing pattern. As the left palm swung forward, facing the ground, she inhaled a long, steady breath. When the next step brought out the right hand, which still faced up, she exhaled audibly. Slowly, she circled the patio, breathing in when the left hand swung forward and exhaling as the right took its place.

After a few minutes, she halted and reversed the hands, turning an open left palm to the sky and directing the right palm toward the ground. I imitated her movements awkwardly. Mind and body stumbled on this unfamiliar path. I found it difficult to keep one hand up and one down while moving forward with focus and balance. *Which hand is supposed to be inhaling here? When do I exhale?* I couldn't shift my focus smoothly back and forth. Feeling the breath in my palms was even harder. OK, she conceded, perhaps the hands aren't *really* breathing, but with practice one can feel the breath of energy flowing through "power points" in the palms, she insisted. According to ancient Chinese teachings, both the palms and the soles of the feet contain energy points that can draw in "chi"—the life force—or release stale energy from the body. Some forms of Chinese medical practice suggest that we can enhance health by circulating energy through these points. "Breathing" through the hands or feet is believed to clear blockages in energy channels that run up and down the body.

In the days that followed, I practiced integrating these concepts into fitness walks. The motions became playful when I increased the pace to an aerobic level and tried to "breathe" through my palms without drawing the attention of passersby in the neighborhood. Instead of holding my hands in soft fists as I usually do for workouts, I turned one wrist up and the other down, opening the fingers just enough to give the energy room to flow. "In-two-three-four," I counted as I imagined energy from the earth rising into my cupped palm. "Out-two-three-four," I exhaled, releasing tired emotions to the sky. It made me smile. I felt silly, like I was holding a secret in the palms of my cupped hands. No observer would know I was moving energy with nothing more than a strong imagination and a steady breath.

But breath *is* energy—pure and simple. Both athletes and meditators learn this truth when they discover the power of deep, conscious breathing. And breath is laughter as well. As you make a "whole coin" investment in walking workouts, a playful attitude enables you to explore the world of mindful movement with freedom and a great deal of pleasure. Fill your lungs with laughter, and be creative in your approach to ideas that seem strange to you. Create imaginary nostrils. Breathe through the hands. Draw energy through the feet. Inhale to the belly and feel the abdomen expand as fresh air massages the energy center below the navel. Allow curiosity to guide your explorations.

"To learn something really new is not a matter of planning or thinking and analyzing. What is required is a clearing or emptying of the mind and the heart so that we can listen in a deep and new way," advise meditation teachers Joseph Goldstein and Jack Kornfield in *Seeking the Heart of Wisdom*. "The willingness to empty ourselves and then seek our true nature is an expression of great and courageous love."[9]

Conscious breathing initiates a natural rhythm of emptying, opening, and finding new ways to love ourselves. Each breath weaves through a multitude of levels to clear a path to greater aliveness that is both physical and symbolic. To empty ourselves with each exhalation sweeps the body of toxins and makes room for inspiration—for the nourishment of fresh air and new information. As you practice making breath awareness a component of your walking workouts, remind yourself that athletes and spiritual seekers alike regard this most basic function of life as the instrument of its highest attainments. Use it to enrich your appreciation of the energy source provided for you at birth. When you breathe with awareness, each breath unites you with the power of life that surrounds and sustains you.

# From Sole to Soul . . .

*Jitterbug Breath:* In Tom Robbins's playful novel *Jitterbug Perfume,* two age-defying characters travel the course of human history after discovering that "a funny way of breathing" brings immortality. The magic that carries them across a dozen normal life spans comes from breathing air in and out of the body in a seamless flow.

Inhale and exhale follow one another in a circular pattern "like a serpent swallowin' its own tail. When they brought air into their bodies, they visualized suckin' in as much energy and vitality as possible; when they expelled air, they visualized blowin' out all the staleness and flatness inside o' them."[10]

It makes an entertaining story and a playful case for the power of good breathing. Perhaps it can't guarantee eternal youth, but as a focusing device for spirited walking, "jitterbug breathing" delivers the miracle of mindfulness that prolongs awareness of the present.

After a warm-up walk, loosen shoulders, hips, and ankles with a few gentle rotations. Begin walking at a pace that will take you into your aerobic workout zone. While breathing through either the nose or mouth, imagine that every exhalation flows out of the body in a gentle arc. As the exhalation ends, imagine the air looping back with the inhalation. Make the circle seamless so that the breath slides smoothly across the pause that usually occurs at the end of an exhale.

Keep the inhale and exhale deep and even, giving each half of the cycle equal time. Guide the pattern by counting steps. Try to extend the breath so that you have three or four steps to each phase—"in-two-three; out-two-three," like a rolling hoop. This exercise is not as simple as it seems. It demands mental focus. The moment your attention slides, the circle will sag into an oval. The in-and-out rhythm becomes uneven. Circle back with the focus and start again.

Try this breathing pattern in short segments during your walks as an intense focusing practice. See if you can maintain the circle breath for two minutes. What about five minutes? When you discover how difficult it can be to focus for even five minutes, you may wonder how you manage to achieve anything in your life. You may also appreciate why our lives often feel stressful and hectic. Our minds constantly chase after this thought or that. Physical exercise provides a mirror of our daily lives and lets us see just how difficult it is to be truly aware, giving full attention to one thing at a time.

If you breathe through the mouth, you may find that "jitterbug breath" leaves your mouth drier than usual. Carry a water bottle you can attach to your belt or find a route with a water fountain, especially in hot weather.

*Inspirational Sprints:* A sprint is a short, all-out effort that asks you to move as fast as you can. Sprints are wonderful for increasing fitness levels because they briefly push you beyond the exertion you've grown comfortable with. By making sprints an occasional feature of your exercise routine, you will gradually raise your comfort zone.

Give yourself at least thirty minutes for this exercise. If possible, go to a track or find a route where you can mentally mark off a distance similar to the track's four-hundred-meter lap. You'll be doing several laps of alternating sprints and recovery, using the breath for energy and focus.

Before you begin the all-out effort of a sprint, it's important to be thoroughly warmed up. When you have finished your warm-up, walk one lap at a pace that you'd call "moderate." It should be just brisk enough to begin to elevate your heart rate. Focus on establishing a deep rhythmic breathing pattern, drawing each breath into the belly so the abdomen expands.

After one lap, you'll probably be ready to move a bit faster. Keep breathing in the same manner, drawing air into the belly, as you push your effort to a level you consider "somewhat hard." When your attention wanders or you begin to tire, focus on your breathing. Count your steps as you inhale and exhale with steady control. Be firm and clear in your commitment. Maintain this pace for three-fourths of the lap. Now, sprint to the finish line. Pick up your feet. Pump your arms. Give it your best effort for the final one hundred meters of the lap. And remember to breathe! Focus on deep, energizing breaths to carry you through any resistance and over the finish line.

Follow the "sprint" lap with a recovery lap at a moderate pace, continuing the practice of focusing on the breath. The pattern looks like this:

A. One lap at "moderate" effort and walking speed

B. Three-fourths lap at "somewhat hard" effort and speed

C. One-fourth lap at "sprint" or "hard" effort and speed

Repeat the cycle at least twice. Do a third set if you have time. Each repetition will lead you deeper into a team effort shared by body and mind. It asks you to invest both sides of the mental-physical coin. Use the breath as a vehicle for listening respectfully to the body. Let it guide you past idle distractions. Be mindful of the body's reactions as you ask for increased effort. And give yourself a mental high-five when you finish. A good workout is something to acknowledge.

# CHAPTER 6

~

# *Daily Walks*

## STEPPING UP THE COMMITMENT

The road between the village of San Felipe del Agua and the central plaza of the Mexican city of Oaxaca runs just outside the wall of an apartment compound where I once spent a month. I said my goal was to study Spanish, but mostly I needed a vacation. More than lessons, I wanted casual chats over *café con leche* at the sidewalk cafés that border Oaxaca's colorful square.

I looked forward to trips into the countryside, to days of prowling the archaeological ruins of Monte Albán and stroking the lanolin-soft texture of hand-woven rugs in

Teotitlán del Valle. I wanted to wrap myself in the restorative mantle of observer, released for a time from the roles and responsibilities I wear at home. Here, all that was required of me was to get from my lodgings to the center of town four miles away. *"No problema,"* I was assured. Buses pass the gate every thirty minutes or so.

"So long, I'm off to catch the bus," I announced as I headed out on the first mornings. I stood at the gate, surrounded by lush sprays of pink and purple bougainvillea, facing north to await my transportation. Sometimes it came just as promised. More often it did not. On those days, I'd shift from one foot to the other and glare in impatience at my watch. Well-designed plans rolled into beads of perspiration and pooled in angry splotches on my shirt. I felt helpless and betrayed. Gone, my *"no problema"* holiday. Daily, my frustration deepened.

It took perhaps two weeks for me to hit on an alternative. "So long," I'd say as I stuffed a map and hat into a shoulder bag. "I'm off to the plaza." Then I'd head out the gate, pass the bougainvillea, and start walking. If the bus came, I flagged it. If it didn't, I'd walk down the street past the cluster of school buildings where children pointed at my watch and asked the time. I cut through the park where young lovers nuzzled amid a morning bloom of bath soap and aftershave.

Beyond the park, I'd reach the neighborhood market where mounds of warm *pan dulce* perfumed the air. "What can I get you?" vendors would call from behind displays of golden papayas and buckets of elegant white calla lilies. On the curb, Zapotec women in traditional shawls sat beside baskets they had filled in the dark of early morning with the handmade staple of Oaxacan meals. "Tortillas?" they entreated as I passed.

In just over an hour, I'd reach the *zócalo*, the central plaza where shoe-shine boys and balloon vendors maintained brisk businesses. Some days, mariachis serenaded at noon from the gazebo at the center. Their notes collided with the amplified speeches of demonstrators camped before government offices to protest pay scales for teachers or working conditions for laborers.

At a sidewalk café, I'd sip a coffee and let the rhythm of the walk ripple through my day, spacing out thoughts and expectations. Gradually the pattern expanded my sense of beginnings and endings. By the time I packed my bags to leave Oaxaca, I had come to regard capricious bus schedules as a high point of my vacation. They had delivered me to a truth I'd forgotten: discovery doesn't depend on the bus. Exploration begins with an attitude, not with a location.

Daily walks make explorers of us all, particularly when we bring awareness to the path. When walking becomes an integrated part of life, a routine as automatic and vital as brushing teeth or recycling yesterday's paper, it introduces patterns that fortify body, mind, and spirit. As with any new habit, creating a spirited walking practice requires a willingness to try something new and the determination to stick with it long enough to make a fair evaluation. It may mean starting over again and again until you slip comfortably into a new self-image. As you come to identify yourself as a walker, you embark on a path of discovery and well-being. As you bring mental focus to your route, you move toward wholeness.

Keep reminding yourself that with thirty minutes of mindful walking you can satisfy the most frequently recommended daily minimum requirements for both exercise and meditation. From the outset, the combination offers an attractive efficiency. Stay with it and you'll discover a ritual of health and wholeness that deepens the value of physical exercise. Medical researcher Herbert Benson reports that athletes who focus awareness on the breath or on a repeated word while exercising achieve the relaxation of the "runners' high" faster than those who do not.[1] He found that simply repeating the words *in* and *out* mentally with the breath while walking reduces anxiety, increases energy, and delivers many of the benefits of traditional meditation. Spiritual teacher and medical adviser Deepak Chopra considers daily meditation such a powerful tool for stilling internal turbulence and creating clarity that he makes it part of the very first principle in *The Seven Spiritual Laws of Success.*[2]

Meanwhile, medical researchers have amassed convincing evidence that physical exercise provides the greatest health benefits when it's done almost daily. A 1996 U.S. surgeon general report concluded that thirty minutes of exercise at a level sufficient to burn a minimum of 150 calories a day, or 1,000 calories a week, produces significant health benefits.[3] For most people, thirty minutes of brisk walking daily meets the surgeon general's prescription for reducing the risk of heart disease, diabetes, hypertension, weight gain, colon cancer, depression, and loss of bone mass.

Walking at a slower pace provides significant mental benefits, and certainly contributes to physical well-being, especially for people who do not exercise regularly. But the surgeon general's report advises that then you walk at a pace that does not elevate heart rate, you'll need to walk longer in order to burn the recommended number of exercise calories daily.

Current research targets a weekly expenditure of 1,000 to 1,500 calories through exercise as a baseline for extending life spans and enhancing physical fitness. An average walker can satisfy the goal with ten to fifteen miles of walking per week—just three miles a day, five days a week. Both meditation and exercise enrich life most profoundly when they are incorporated into the values and patterns that shape your days. The secret of your success lies in taking daily steps toward mental and physical well-being.

## IN THE HABIT

"The hard part is acquiring the habit," acknowledges attorney Charles Porter.[4] "It has to be made a rigid part of your daily schedule." Every weekday and frequently on Saturdays, Porter walks two and a half miles from his Oregon home to his law office. His usual path leads through a neighborhood park, past the high school soccer field, and into the heart of town. He sets a brisk aerobic pace, starting out before daylight on winter mornings. Along the route, he sometimes prepares for court. He might mentally rehearse an opening statement or closing comments to get the feel of the words he will speak. More often, he simply clears his head.

"Sometimes I like having an empty mind and just breathing and letting things occur," he says. Although he carries a notepad in a pocket to capture flashes of inspiration, most of the time he focuses his attention on the subtle variations in the color of the hills or the changing texture of the trees as seasons move across his route. Walking became part of Porter's daily life when he returned from two terms in the U.S. House of Representatives and looked for quiet space in a busy schedule. In walking, he found a practical respite from telephones and legal technicalities. Since then, the walks have paved a daily transition between personal and professional roles, between seasons of the year and cycles of life. For thirty-five years, the ritual has offered exercise and peace of mind. Out of it has evolved a clear code of ethics that governs Porter's excursions: leave headsets and cell phones behind. ("Quiet time is too precious for distractions.") Reflect and observe as you walk. ("It is lonely but lovely.") Exert yourself. ("Time yourself and try to improve.") Persevere regardless of weather. ("Carry an umbrella in a knapsack.")

"It's part of the quality of my life," says Porter, who at seventy-eight shows no signs of cutting back his walks, his full-time law practice, or his regular squash matches. "It's very handy. When you arrive at work, you are ready. You just have to build it in to your life, and then you do it. You have to be iron-willed, and you can't make excuses for yourself. Then it's not so hard."

But discipline is never simple, whether it supports a meditation practice or fitness workouts. We resist it almost automatically, pushing against the notion of controls and balking at the thought of rules. Somehow discipline sounds harsh and punitive—but it doesn't need to be. It really only means making conscious choices. It means being aware and responsible for decisions and behaviors that control us. Isn't that what we really want? If you decide to make daily walks part of your life, try to suspend harsh demands and self-criticism as you establish a new routine. How many tries did it take you to learn to tie a shoelace? To catch a ball? To write your own name? Who can remember? What remains today is the skill acquired with those repetitions. That's what makes the word *practice* so appropriate for a spiritual pursuit. Practice recognizes the role of repetition in shaping new abilities. It describes a regular pattern of behavior, a custom, a habit, a reliable ritual that gives continuity to our lives. Practice absolves us from expectations of perfection or from the erratic excesses of "binge" exercise.

"The key word for our time is *practice*. We have all the light we need, we just need to put it into practice," advised Peace Pilgrim, a woman who dropped her own identity and put aside the comforts of contemporary life to travel the United States on foot for twenty-eight years in an active prayer for peace.[5] Her steps were a demonstration of her belief that world peace begins with personal peace. When we fail to find inner peace, it is not because we can't but because we do not try, she maintained. "There is no glimpse of the light without walking the path."[6]

One way to assist yourself in creating a regular walking meditation practice is to sign an agreement with yourself. Health educators say that written contracts hold up much

# *Side* *Lines*

## TAKING IT ON THE SHIN

When walkers pick up the pace or frequency of their workouts, they place unfamiliar demands on the body. It's not unusual to experience a little muscle stiffness during an initial period of adjustment.

The muscles along the front of the lower leg may be the first to raise a complaint. These muscles get a lot of use during walking—they lift and lower the toes. Unfortunately, in a sedentary lifestyle, this specialized muscle experiences few demands—beyond pushing down the gas pedal.

Stretching and strengthening the lower leg muscles can help relieve shin discomfort as you build endurance for longer walks. You can actually strengthen lower leg muscles while watching television or talking on the phone. Simply cross your legs and write the alphabet with the toe of the raised leg. Switch legs and repeat.

Before a walk, loosen ankles and shins with a few foot rotations to get blood flowing. Put your weight on one leg and raise the other foot a few inches off the ground. Rotate the toe of the raised foot to make half a dozen circles in each direction.

If soreness continues during your walk, take a break to rotate the ankles a few more times and release muscle tension. At the end of your walk, stretch the muscles you have used and build increased strength in calves and ankles with heel lifts. Stand on a flat surface, feet together. Lift the heels as high as you can, stretching up on your toes. Hold the stretch a few seconds and then lower gently. Try not to let the weight of the body drop on the heel. Repeat the lift up to twenty times, holding a few seconds at the top each time. Make the movement slow and controlled to protect the complex mechanisms of the foot and ankle.

If you are familiar with the child's pose from hatha yoga and have no problems with your knees, try that position to stretch and relax the shins before you go to bed at night. The child's pose is a forward curl that gets its name from the posture of sleeping infants. Start in a kneeling position on hands and knees. The feet should be extended behind you with the toes pointed back. Gently lower the buttocks toward the heels. Go only as far as is comfortable. The weight of your body should create a good stretch on the front of the lower leg. Relax and hold the pose for a minute.

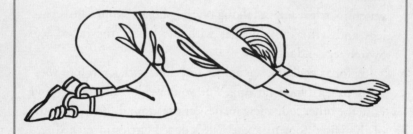

### SHIN STRETCH

Be patient. Usually, the shin discomfort that walkers experience is the result of underdeveloped muscles rather than injury. When you develop a daily walking practice, recognize that it may take a little time to strengthen this part of your body.

better than good intentions even when you are your own judge and jury.[7] Create a personal contract by deciding what goals you are willing to set for the next month. Be clear and reasonable as you outline an agreement:

- How many days will you walk each week? Every day? Every other day?

- How many minutes will you walk each time?

- Will you schedule a longer walk on weekends?

- When will you walk? Be specific about scheduling the walk into your day.

- Where will you walk?

- Will you walk alone or with another person?

- Will you join a weekly walking group for added motivation?

- How will you incorporate meditation or mental focus into your walks?

- Will you click off the distraction of TV when you walk on a treadmill?

Write out your agreement. For best results, you need to see it in black and white before you sign it. Now decide how you will reward yourself for meeting the terms of the contract. Perhaps you promise yourself a new pair of shoes at the end of the month. What about a walking stick for summer hikes? Or a book of daily inspiration to read before you walk? Maybe you'd prefer a bouquet of roses, a gift of love for keeping your word.

If you really want to boost your odds of getting those roses or walking shoes, seek assistance. Get a friend, your partner, a neighbor, or coworker to read your contract and support you in keeping up the effort to create a new habit. Tell this person what kind of assistance you'd like. Do you want daily reminders or a phone call once a week to ask how the program is going?

In recent years, I've depended on three friends to help me pursue dreams. We meet one morning a week to check in on events of the previous week. Then we spend a few minutes in silence, writing individual goals for the days ahead. The weekly act of focusing on two or three clear outcomes that we want in our personal, professional, or social lives helps us clarify our own intentions. Reading them aloud to one another sets up a pattern of feedback and support. Don't underestimate the power of the written word. A personal contract has the force to carry you to your goals.

## A BOOK OF MIRACLES

The goal that carries Mari Messer out for walks in the chill of an Ohio winter is the search for a daily miracle. Each walk affords an opportunity to reaffirm the magic of life. One day last winter it was the tiny tadpole she glimpsed beneath the ice of a frozen pond. Its bulging eyes peered up at her as she stopped at the edge of her walking trail, caught by the unexpected movement. In the midst of winter, it seemed symbolic. A miracle, she says. An affirmation of renewal and spirit amid the snow and barren branches.

Another day it was the tiny blue flower, no larger than a pearl, that she saw in the grass of a golf course. A bloom so small and out of place that she marveled at its tenacity and its dedication to purpose. Like the tadpole, it gained recognition in the book of miracles where she records her discoveries. "Whatever stands out as a small miracle of the day goes into my journal, and it's almost always something I observe on my walks," she says.[8] "It can be the tiniest experience. I open all my senses when I walk and try to notice what is there. That's the way you enrich your walking, the mindfulness."

Each year Mari selects a special appointment book in which to record a daily miracle. Day by day, she fills it with evidence of life's wonder and mystery. A public relations consultant, she schedules time for daily walks just as she schedules client appointments. "There is something so healing about walking in general, and particularly about walking in nature. It's a spiritual practice in that I do it mindfully. If you go out with a kind of openness, you get the benefit. It's like a minivacation from whatever bothers you, and when you come back, you feel refreshed."

Usually she walks alone, making her walks a silent practice of awareness and attentiveness to nature. "You aren't really by yourself," she maintains. "The sun and the trees and everything in nature are your walking companions. You can't really have the same intimate connection with them if you are walking with someone else."

It's even harder to make that kind of connection with nature when you can't walk at all. The miracle that Susan

Freisinger seeks is the strength to take a single step. Four years after an automobile accident broke her neck and damaged her spinal cord, Susan sits in a wheelchair and strolls through memories to recapture the magic of walks she can no longer take. "For me, walking was the rhythm of my life," she says. "Throughout my life, I have meditated a lot. Part of my meditation was walking." She pauses to let her cells retrieve the rolling rhythm of a stroll, to sense the earth beneath her feet. Slowly she lifts her arm and circles a hand in front of her, carving smooth rotations in the air. Walking felt like that, she says. Like a cycle. A clear, steady rhythm that connected head and legs. A pattern that linked the soul and the earth. "Now, since I can't do that, I feel stagnant. I feel a disconnectedness to the world. I feel cut off from myself."[9]

Her words plant a miracle in the air. Her clarity ignites a candle of awareness. Each step . . . each day . . . each tree . . . each hand. Each one, a miracle.

## STEPPING UP AWARENESS

If you've been experimenting with the exercises suggested in previous chapters of this book, you're already walking with increased mindfulness. One thing you're probably keenly aware of is just how challenging fitness walking can be when you exercise both muscles and mind. To achieve health benefits, you may have found that you need to walk faster or longer. To develop a state of mindfulness, you've had to rein in random thoughts. Both are forms of training that take practice and patience. Initially, you may hear some protests when you increase the workouts and move toward a daily practice of aerobic walking meditation. If you experience muscle soreness, warm up thoroughly before pushing to an aerobic walking pace. Take time to stretch at the end of workouts. Be consistent and committed to your goals without making unreasonable demands on yourself. Listen carefully and respectfully, knowing that you are on a fitness course that brings mental training into step with physical exercise.

"Training the mind, as an athlete tunes and trains his body, is one of the primary aims of all forms of meditation," asserts psychologist Lawrence LeShan, author of *How to Meditate*, a primer of meditation practices. "This is one of the basic reasons that this discipline increases efficiency in everyday life."[10] Just as regular exercise strengthens the body's physical functioning, daily meditation enhances its mental powers of concentration, focus, and clarity. It makes no difference whether that practice takes place on neighborhood sidewalks or in the cushioned silence of an ashram.

Author Jack Kornfield relates a wonderful story about his early training in Zen Buddhism. When he joined a monastic community, he found himself burdened with domestic chores that interfered with time to sit in silent meditation. Dissatisfaction clattered through his thoughts as he carried out the tasks he'd been assigned. Eventually, he began to doubt the teacher he had chosen to follow. He saw flaws wherever he looked. He went to the teacher with his concerns. All this activity, he said, this coming and going, the endless distractions, it leaves no time for meditation. No time to learn what he had come for. The teacher listened attentively and responded with a gentle question: "There isn't enough time to be aware?"[11]

The story echoes the message delivered to me on the outskirts of Oaxaca: discovery doesn't depend on the bus. Meditation is an attitude. Meditation is mindfulness, moment to moment. It is not a posture, not a place. It is a constant practice of connecting fully and completely with the present. It is a way of walking through life, seeking to make a conscious choice in everything we do. Ultimately, LeShan says, the path of meditation leads us home. It connects us with parts of ourselves that we have forgotten or been unable to hear in the roar of daily life. It guides us toward a greater sense of wholeness and connection, enabling us to "more fully live the potential of being human" and increasing our ability to give and receive love.

You need not shave your head or practice meditation for a lifetime in order to tap that well of human potential. A newcomer to the weekly meditation circle I attend arrived one evening bearing the benefits of mindfulness in a warm smile. During a difficult time in her personal life, she'd stumbled onto the healing path of walking meditation. In recent weeks, a restless agitation had jarred her sitting meditations. Daily exercise walks had deteriorated into forty-minute assaults of self-criticism and blame as she bumped against the sharp-edged pain of a severed relationship. "When I walked, my mind would go racing around, and I found the things I was thinking weren't good or helpful for me," she told me later. In desperation, she reached for a tool of meditation to silence the accusations that spilled through her head. She turned her focus to a prayer by Saint Francis of Assisi that she had memorized, letting the words fill her mind as she walked:

*Lord, make me an instrument of thy peace.*
*Where there is hatred, let me sow love;*
*Where there is injury, pardon;*
*Where there is doubt, faith;*
*Where there is despair, hope;*
*Where there is darkness, light;*
*Where there is sadness, joy.*
*O divine Master, grant that I may not so much seek*
*To be consoled as to console,*
*To be understood as to understand,*
*To be loved as to love;*
*For it is in giving that we receive;*
*It is in pardoning that we are pardoned;*
*It is in dying [to self] that we are born to eternal life.*[12]

Almost immediately, she stepped into a calming interval, a sense of peace she had been unable to reach by fitness walking or sitting meditation alone. "The combination of exercise and mind-set definitely alters my state of being," she says. Some days, the words set a brisk pace for her feet as she experiments with speed and rhythm. Sometimes she slows to a pensive stroll, adopting the patterns of traditional walking meditation. "It is how I am meditating daily now," she says. "It is training my mind, and I have noticed a difference. It feels right. What my mind is getting now is much more positive than what it was getting before."

Whether you turn to the prayers of spiritual masters or to the visual imagery of athletes as the tools of mental training, you're almost certain to feel some impact as you learn to clear the mind of distracting self-talk. Experiment with a variety of meditation techniques as you walk, trying each device for a week or two so that you let yourself discover its unique benefits. Affirmations help rewrite self-talk. Breathing cleanses the body. Visions tap the power of imagination. Prayers and poems bring inspiration.

Sampling a variety of approaches keeps the process fresh and mentally engaging. My own walks often cycle through an assortment of focusing methods, ranging from affirmation to counting my steps. It makes no difference which I choose, my attention inevitably drifts. In a flash, my mind dashes off to snare some hidden doubt or fear. Like a cat with a catch, it waits on the step of my awareness for me to see this prized discovery. I take a deep breath, give thanks for the reminder, and start again with a word, a phrase, a breath, or an image.

Sometimes I wonder if my eclectic approach is too inclusive and diverse to produce true mindfulness. I worry that my range reveals a lack of discipline. For now, I push the doubts aside with memories of Oaxaca. Daily walks support my commitment to a practice of fitness for body, mind, and spirit. They reflect my dedication to exploration and awareness. I remind myself of the warm delight I encountered in Mexico when I shifted my focus from transportation to destination—I remember the joy I found in the journey, the freedom and connection I encountered when my awareness expanded enough to reveal more than one way to reach the heart of the city.

# From Sole to Soul . . .

*Expect a Miracle:* Daily walks assume a spiritual quality when you set out in search of magic. "What you see is what you get," comedian Flip Wilson used to say, and it's true not only in comedy. When you train yourself to see miracles, they show up often in your life.

With practice, bird-watchers develop keen abilities to spot the subtle differences between species. Golfers learn to follow the arc of a white dot against the sky. Naturalists learn to track animals by detecting minute markings on trees. The same skill and practice enable us to notice the miracles that surround us constantly.

Indoors or out, miracles emerge if we let them. It might be the sunshine that spills from pungent peels of fresh-cut oranges at the juice bar. Perhaps it's the fragment of a song that slips through time and elevator doors to resurrect people or places. Miracles invite us to open our eyes to the simple but unexpected. Nature essayist Terry Tempest Williams tells of the miracle that brought an indoor Christmas tree to life for her one year. The final decorations had just been hung on the tree when a bird flew down the chimney and emerged through the flames of a holiday fire. It circled three times and then perched on the tree, a living ornament.[13]

Make it your goal to locate a miracle the next time you take a walk. Look at your route with fresh eyes, as if you were traveling it for the first time. While you warm up and cool down from the aerobic phase of the walk, look around at your environment for something that captures your imagination and reminds you of life's creativity, humor, or strength.

Be aware of the miracle of your own energy as you travel through a brisk workout. Notice the air, the supporting surface beneath your feet. Simply notice. Expect a miracle and give thanks when you spot one. Perhaps you'll want to make a note of it in your walking log. With practice, you'll gain ease and expertise in spotting the miracles, metaphors, and moments of magic that reward a spirited tracker.

*Gaining Ground on a Treadmill:* One of the biggest obstacles in the path to a daily walking practice appears with a change in the weather. Promises made on a sunny morning disappear when rain dampens enthusiasm. Some people brave the storm and walk in almost any weather. Others pack in their commitment and build a fire.

It could be that your alternative will be to walk indoors. Malls have become popular fitness centers for walkers who turn up early to stride the corridors before stores open. Security, climate-control, and companionship make malls an inviting option. Treadmills offer another choice that keeps you moving when the weather tempts you to slow down. Treadmills may lack scenic appeal, but they make up for it in convenience, effectiveness, and versatility. A study at the Medical College of Wisconsin in Milwaukee confirmed that treadmills beat out other popular exercise machines for efficient calorie burning.[14]

Take advantage of the treadmill's versatility to add variety to your walking routes. If your outdoor workout doesn't include a hill, let a treadmill provide the slope. When you increase the incline of the walking ramp, you boost the effort that you expend while walking, and you strengthen different muscles. It brings balance to your walking practice.

Treadmills also simplify interval workouts that boost your aerobic capacity and walking speed. After a thorough warm-up, increase the belt speed to a pace that puts you in the "somewhat hard" category. Hold that pace for two minutes and then reduce it to a comfortable stroll for two minutes. Repeat the sequence several times, alternating between two-minute segments that you describe as "somewhat hard" walking and "moderate" walking.

Never stop the belt completely or come to a full rest after the hard walking interval. The body recovers best and builds endurance and strength when you keep moving. Cool down gradually at the completion of a workout by slowly reducing the belt speed.

# CHAPTER 7

Yes, I Can!

## MAINTAINING MOTIVATION
## AND CLEARING HURDLES

Early in my enthusiasm for walking, I strode to workouts with the eagerness of an infatuated suitor. Curiosity and discovery propelled me. I couldn't wait to explore every aspect of this new relationship that made me feel so alive. I bought a black plastic sports watch to time my walks. Next came a portable tape player and a recording of up-tempo jazz to lift my mood on foot-dragging days. Before long, I'd found a group of walkers who worked out weekly with a coach. With a newcomer's passion for adventure, I entered track meets for senior athletes and discovered a physical outlet for my love of challenge. Along the way I discovered that physical pursuits succeed or fail on the fitness of mental skills.

On a hot August weekend, four members of my workout group paced nervously at the starting line of a ten-kilometer race and fretted about the heat. We felt the sizzle of nervous energy and questioned the naïveté that had carried us to a neighboring state for a three-day track meet for athletes above the age of thirty-five. At 8:00 A.M. the air already held a stillness that predicted continuation of the weather pattern that had pushed temperatures above 100 degrees for the past two days. With six and two-tenths miles of walking ahead of me, it would be essential to pace myself. But I had a strategy in mind.

Among the walkers gathered for the event, I'd spotted a woman I recognized. Two days before, this woman had passed me in a shorter walk, moving easily ahead when I began to tire in the final minutes. Her steady step won my admiration. Today, I'd let her set my pace. My goal was to let her guide me toward a better racing style. At the starter's command, I held myself back, controlling the adrenaline that bubbled in my veins. *Easy does it,* I reminded myself, as I moved into position at her shoulder. *Calm and steady. Arms relaxed.* I dropped back half a step as the pack spread out.

About fifty participants ranging in age from thirty-five to seventy stretched out along a course that looped through the tree-lined backstreets of a college campus. The woman ahead of me was ten years my senior, a national champion in her age division. My footsteps fell into rhythm with hers. Our arms swung like pendulums in synch, creating a momentum that carried me. If all went well, we'd cross the finish line in just about an hour.

For forty minutes I rode her shoulder. Then slowly the rhythm shifted. My feet lost the beat. My arms fumbled with the pattern. She began to pull ahead. In a flash, despair filled my head: *I can't keep up. It's too hot. What am I doing here?* A mental battle erupted. *Pick up your arms! Push off the toes,* my inner-coach shouted. *I can't. My legs feel heavy. I think I'm dizzy.*

For the next mile, I dodged the attacks of an internal ambush. Through the cross fire, I watched the back I'd set my sights on slowly move ahead. I felt defeated—unable to meet my own goal. *What's the use?* my mind chided. Disappointment blinded me, and I stopped in the middle of the street. *You see,* it taunted. *You couldn't do it. I knew it. This is embarrassing. You were really dumb to try.* Frantically, I searched for rebuttals. Why continue? For me, the race was over. My ego raged at humiliation. *It's in or out,* it snapped angrily. *Get moving or give up.* Stubbornly, I leaned into a head wind of self-criticism and regained my footing on the route.

As I crossed the finish line, the elation of completion erased disappointment. I stepped into the happy camaraderie of women on the other side. We strolled the sidewalks to cool down, wearing our sweat and fatigue with pride. When I'd caught my breath, I approached the woman who'd walked away from me. "How did you do that?" I asked. I wanted to know how she stayed so steady. I wanted to know how she avoided the complaints and resistance that buffet me when I begin to tire. What does she do at that two-thirds point where I always want to stop? What magic keeps her moving?

"Oh," she laughed, "there's no magic. I just start singing 'Yankee Doodle Dandy' to myself."

I stared in stunned amazement. "Yankee Doodle"? I gasped. I couldn't believe it. While I fought a frantic battle with resistance, she stuck a feather in her hat and rode away on the rhythms of a song. Abracadabra. Something flipped in my head. No magic. No mystery. No athletic wizardry. Her secret was nothing more than distraction—like entertaining a child with a key ring.

The mind, I've learned, can be a fussy child, quickly bored and easily distracted. "Yankee Doodle" replaced resistance with entertainment, creating a diversion from the mental temper tantrums that scream, *Why am I doing this?* The stirring battle song of revolutionary soldiers rallies the inner strength of the warrior in sports, as well as war. It leads an internal attack against resistance and self-doubt. I've been singing it gratefully ever since.

## BREAKING THE RESISTANCE BARRIER

There's no escaping encounters with resistance. No matter where we turn, we bump against it. We resist change. We resist boredom. We resist discipline. We resist uncertainty. But there are no breakthroughs without barriers.

Resistance stands at the door to discovery. The power to live fully in the present, free from past regrets and future fears, lies in learning to recognize resistance as simply one of the many choices available to a resourceful mind.

Most often, resistance arises from fear. Fear of pain, fear of failure, fear of boredom, fear of commitment, fear of crowds, fear of isolation, fear of abandonment, fear of responsibility, fear of criticism—it stops us from exploring and risking. Philosopher Alan Watts said that fear is simply the other side of freedom.[1] Turn it over and we can get what we want. Poet Rainer Maria Rilke compared our deepest fears to the raging dragons of fairy tales that turn into princesses when befriended.[2]

But you can't blame fear for every clash with resistance on your walking path. Sometimes resistance is as simple and inescapable as inertia. Sometimes resistance presents the voice of reason, the wisdom of moderation. Whatever the source or form that resistance takes, it creates a powerful presence. If you've ever abandoned a resolution, dropped out of an exercise program, or given up a goal, you've been blocked by the resistance barrier. If you've experimented with the exercises and aerobic paces suggested in the *From Sole to Soul* sections of this book, you've bumped against resistance. Mental training and a playful attitude can soften its impact.

Just as weight training helps develop healthy muscles and aerobic training builds a strong heart, mental training empowers the mind. Breaking through the resistance barrier calls for focus and mindfulness. Mindfulness sounds simple but often isn't. It requires that you stay awake and fully conscious of your actions, feelings, and thoughts. It means steering clear of the "automatic pilot" that propels us through life in a stupor. The ability to stay present and aware enables you to spot resistance quickly and move it aside or find another route to your goal. A daily walking practice provides a steady source of opportunities for practicing mental skills that can move you beyond resistance and into freedom.

Songs, chants, affirmations, visual images, waltzes, breath awareness, a meaningful word—all have the power to strengthen your willpower when resistance dares you to take the day off. They silence the temptation to cut walks short. They carry you through the urge to pull back every time you attempt to walk farther or faster than usual. The first step in getting beyond resistance comes in learning its patterns and habits. Watch for it in these predictable guises:

*Walker's Block:* Often the first obstacle you encounter in a fitness program is the law of inertia: a body at rest remains at rest. In fact, a body at rest *resists* motion. Just getting out the door triggers resistance. Expect this opposition. Know it will happen. Once the body gets moving, you can relax a little. It takes less effort to maintain motion.

To minimize Walker's Block, try scheduling walks at the same time each day to create an habitual pattern. Write down walk times on a calendar to increase visibility and commitment. Set out walking clothes before you go to bed at night. Pack your gym bag if you take clothes with you to work. Arrange to meet someone and walk together. Just do it.

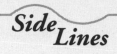
# Side Lines

## THE JOY OF COMPLETION

Even experienced athletes face battles with resistance, as runner-philosopher George Sheehan demonstrated in this eloquent essay written for *Runner's World* at a time when he was also battling the cancer that claimed his life in 1993.[3]

As I neared the two-mile mark of a 5-mile race in Ocean County Park, New Jersey, I was running dead last, 107th in a field of 107.

At that point, a park ranger who was working as a course monitor called out to me. "How are you doing?" he asked.

"The best I can," I panted.

For me, doing the best I can is routine, but being last is an unusual experience.

Once, when I ran in a national championships in my 40s, I was lapped by the entire field. But not since then had I held the position that defines the end of the race.

There was no question that I was last. I turned around several times to be certain. Surrounded by silence, I felt as if I were alone on a training run in the woods.

About 200 yards ahead, my friend Jason was holding his steady pace. Beyond him I could intermittently see a small group of stragglers winding through the tree-lined streets. Each of us wrestled with our private struggle, trying to maintain the level of exertion a 5-mile race demands.

Not only did I have to work hard, but I had to fight off temptation as well. This was a two-loop course, and as I neared the halfway point, dropping out seemed like a wonderful alternative. We all know what this feels like. On loop courses, where the opportunity presents itself at every lap to pack it in, we can't help but have at least a transient impulse to call it quits.

But within a few strides the thought passed, and I knew if I started into the second loop it wouldn't come again. It never did.

The philosopher William Barrett . . . writes that the runner who's lapped by the entire field but nevertheless tortures himself to keep going is "more admirable than the victor we crown." Faith and belief and prayer—these subjects dominate Barrett's writing. And for him, the ritual—in this instance, the race—provides a discipline and gives our lives meaning.

I had a mile to go. Jason was beginning to come back to me. Both of us in this hour were finding our meaning in apparently meaningless suffering. Both were sending a wordless prayer to a higher power. Both were believing that our running made the best statement of who we are.

In the last 20 yards, still trying to do my very best, I finally caught Jason and sprinted by him. Beyond the finish line, where I lay gasping on the ground, Jason came by to congratulate me. Then I heard someone say, "The best race of the day was for last place."

He didn't know the half of it.

*Two-Thirds Tedium:* This is the voice that whines, *Haven't we done enough now?* It arises out of boredom. It wants a change. Sometimes it worries about fatigue. *I'm tired,* it says. *This hurts my knee.* Pay attention and listen carefully. Is the fear of injury legitimate? Is the resistance really fear of not keeping up, of failing, of looking foolish, of getting sweaty?

Try a mental diversion. Focus on a song or affirmation or meditation tool for five minutes, then check on the pain. Is it worse? Did it disappear? Should you stop or slow down? Be reasonable. Make a conscious, informed choice. Often physical distress disappears when body and mind work out together. The active use of mental focusing techniques during exercise has been shown to increase muscle efficiency.[4] Literally, your thoughts determine how hard your body has to work.

My walks invariably seem to get tougher at the two-thirds mark, regardless of the distance I'm going. Usually that's when I begin to feel tired or bored. My brain gets restless and looks for something else to do. It dredges up aches and pains and complaints—anything that might create change. With practice, I've learned to interrupt the cycle with a pattern of my own: Take a breath. Realign body posture. Pick a focus. Often my first choice is simply to start counting. In-two-three-four, out-two-three-four, paying attention to my breath. With the change, my awareness returns to the present. My body feels lighter, my steps easier.

*Upgrades:* Put a slope in my path and I can count on repercussions. The extra effort of a hill guarantees that my momentum and mental focus will bog down. Every ounce of me grumbles in protest.

"The best way out is always through," the poet Robert Frost advised, proposing a head-on approach to problems.[5] When confronted by the problem of an upgrade, I swing back. Literally, I pump my arms harder, shorten my stride, and move with brisk steps up the hill. Often I focus on the three-step waltz rhythm of *The Blue Danube,* chanting "yes-I-can, yes-I-can" as I glide forward. At the top, I delight in a sense of victory. Small successes give me confidence to tackle bigger challenges.

*Speed Bumps:* When you speed up your walking pace to an aerobic workout level, you can expect to encounter objections. Target heart rates make us work a little harder than usual. Hang on and you'll pass through the resistance, like emerging from a layer of turbulent air on an airplane flight.

Take time to warm up thoroughly before pushing to aerobic levels, and you'll create a smoother, safer transition from a resting heart rate to a working one. Still, even at a slow, steady rate of increase, you're likely to encounter mental turbulence every time you press for greater effort. Often this is a signal that you're reaching an aerobic workout level that will bring healthy benefits. Use mental focusing to maintain the pace and keep your progress steady.

By learning to identify the patterns of resistance that can push you off course, you take a huge step toward achieving fitness goals. An acquaintance who owns a fitness club observes the impact of resistance daily on unprepared exercisers. She watches new members launch vigorous workout programs with ambitious goals. They jump on the step machine and immediately push for full exertion. They huff and puff for five awful minutes and then announce that it's boring. They switch to something else. They don't hang on through the turbulence of warm-up. They never settle into an exercise groove.

"On the StairMaster, at fifteen minutes I hit my pace," this friend says. "Everything clicks. People who only exercise for ten minutes never find that spot. All they are doing is the hard part."[6] Experienced exercisers recognize that there are ups and downs in every workout. They know it takes a few minutes to get beyond the sluggishness of start-up. They've learned that if they stick with it, they usually feel better at the end of a workout than they do before they start.

Mental focusing can motivate you to hang on through the resistance that arises on every walk. And the benefits don't stop with motivation. Researchers at the University of Massachusetts found that walkers who practiced mental focusing techniques during walks returned from exercise with significantly less anxiety and negativity than walkers who allowed their minds to wander.[7] No matter what form of focus you select, your practice strengthens mental agility and enables you to put aside the distractors that drain energy from dreams.

## GOOD CENTS

When Cheryl Brozovic measured a two-mile course in her neighborhood and started walking after work, she watched the scales for motivation. Each pound that dropped her closer to her goal boosted her commitment to exercise. By the time she lost forty-five pounds, she didn't need the scales to keep her going. She had picked up a passion, as well as a hobby. She'd become a coin collector.

At first, it was the traditional promise of good luck that prompted Cheryl to stop for a penny on her walking path. Pretty soon, she was depositing the pennies in a jar at home. "Can't have too much good luck," she reasoned, as the collection grew. The coins were fun—an entertaining extra to her exercise program.

As her fitness increased, Cheryl extended her territory. A practice that started with two miles a day stretched to five-mile walks on weekdays and longer distances on weekends. Her sense of adventure kept pace. She trekked in Nepal and hiked a scenic gorge in Greece. She walked a marathon. After each experience, she returned to the familiar streets around her Michigan home with a fresh eye and renewed appreciation for the social, physical, and emotional value of walking.

For twelve years she followed her daily practice, walking through corporate parking lots and industrial areas near her home. And she continued to pick up pennies until her good-luck jar spilled over. She counted the coins and put $268.24 into a new winter coat. Now the jar is filling again.

"Walking has become so much a part of my life now that I just don't feel right if I don't exercise," Cheryl says.[8] These days motivation comes not only from pounds and pennies but also from the compliments she collects along her route. Neighbors, delivery people, commuters, and store employees all recognize her as "the neighborhood walker." They stop

149

to ask how many miles she's walking today, how many miles she's walked since she started. "People tell me they see me all the time and they know they should get out and do the same thing. That makes me feel good. I like to think I am inspiring people to do something good for themselves."

Sometimes people ask to walk with her. Most of the time she declines, citing scheduling problems. But it's really time alone that she's protecting. Time to clear her head. Even after she fought off an attacker, she has maintained a solitary practice. The threat brought mindfulness and focus. It taught her to pay attention to the present. "I could not let myself be a prisoner," she says. "I learned to be more aware."

Threats have a powerful way of boosting awareness. They alert us to the risks of absentmindedness—of living or walking without focus. When I changed jobs a few years ago, the threat of financial loss filled me with uncertainty. As I faced my fear, I turned to affirmations of prosperity for reassurance. "All my needs are met with abundance and ease," I recited on daily walks.

On weekend walks with my husband, I began to envy the frequency with which he found pennies in the street. He picked them up with exclamations of glee. "A penny! I found a penny," he'd announce. His delight seemed excessive to me. All this for a single cent? But the pattern continued— him picking up pennies, me reciting affirmations for abundance and prosperity. Eventually, the challenge drew me in. I wanted to find pennies, too. I turned my focus to the street.

Mindfulness paid off. After walks, I'd drop the pennies into a basket of "found treasures"—rocks, shells, beads, and curiosities that I've collected over the years. Now coins slipped into the assortment, another treasure lying in my path. Gradually, their value compounded until I purchased a new attitude. "Thank you," I say now when I pick up a penny. "Thank you for the abundance that lies in my path. My life is rich and blessed."

These coins are no longer small change. As I began to celebrate pennies as symbols of the abundant resources in my life, each discovery reminded me to keep my eyes open to all possibilities—to be grateful for small blessings as well as big ones. They constantly expand my definition of wealth. Each deepens my commitment to mindfulness. If I can't see a penny, what else might I be missing?

Day after day, the metaphor converts my scarcity fears to gratitude for options. Each coin brings delight and reassurance. It pays benefits in triplicate. First, each sets off the thrill of an unexpected gift, a treasure-hunt success. Next comes the warmth of gratitude. When my basket of blessings overflows, the coins spill into a celebration, contributing to a dinner out or to "fun money" for a vacation.

## MOTIVATION AT YOUR FEET

By itself, one penny doesn't buy much. But a penny a day is a very different matter. These pennies can add up to a convincing asset. The same compounding of value occurs when you build a collection of motivational tools. The more techniques you pick up, the more options you'll have when you need a boost. Variety brings diversion and fun, the foundation of athletic motivation.

Motivation is what gets you off the sofa and out the door. It keeps you moving through the resistance you encounter during walks. Motivation thrives on creativity and imagination. Health and weight may prompt you to begin a fitness walking program, but start-up impetus quickly fades, no matter how many resolutions you make. Unless your walks bring mental, spiritual, and physical rewards, you aren't likely to travel far.

Previous chapters have exposed my eclectic approach to motivation. Tigers delight me. "Yankee Doodle" entertains me. Affirmations calm me. Focused breathing clears my head. All of them lead to the same goal: they connect my mind and body in the present moment. They replace fragmentation with wholeness. They reawaken awareness and energy. Let your imagination create personalized motivational tools based on the techniques introduced in previous chapters. When you need a fresh surge of energy, dip into this list of additional suggestions to support and strengthen your commitment to a spirited walking practice:

*Buff Up Your Walker Image:* Surround yourself with walking images and inspiration. Read an issue of *Walking* magazine to pick up training techniques and helpful tips for walkers at all levels. Health and fitness magazines let you become part of a vast community of athletes dedicated to well-being. Books and essays about walking by dedicated walkers such as Hal Borland, Ruth Rudner, Colin Fletcher, or Henry David Thoreau draw you into a world of walkers. Check the resource guide at the end of this book for additional suggestions.

Make a fitness collage with pictures and motivational messages cut from magazines. Collages create visible goals. They identify an attitude, a sense of vitality and health, a walking vacation, a trekking adventure, and other goals that motivate you to walk regularly.

*Fascinating Rhythm:* When nothing else gets my spirit moving, music is magic. The steady beat of an invigorating rhythm lifts my soles and my soul faster than anything else. Studies indicate that I'm not alone. Research shows that music motivates exercisers to work out harder and longer, especially when people choose music they enjoy and songs that match their pace.[9]

But tape players are controversial. Many people warn that they diminish a walker's awareness of traffic and other safety hazards. Meditational walkers often prefer silence. Use music only in areas where you feel safe, and always keep one ear free so that you remain aware of sounds around you. Let music be an occasional treat, saved for days when you need an extra nudge. Because spirited walking requires mental focus, select instrumental music only. Vocal music is distracting, but you can repeat affirmations or focus on the breath quite effectively with the steady beat of instrumental music in the background.

*Have a Heart:* Heart-rate monitors lend another technological boost to motivation. Basically, the monitors are an expensive alternative to simply taking your pulse, but they are easier to interpret and a lot more fun.

The most accurate monitors consist of a band worn around the chest and a wristwatch that picks up a heartbeat signal transmitted from the chest band. A simple glance at the dial gives you an instantaneous reading of your heart rate. Research with walkers has shown that heart rate monitors increase interest and pace.[10] They are available at athletic stores and many discount stores with prices beginning at about one hundred dollars.

*Skip a Beat:* Sometimes resistance comes as a premature warning of fatigue. It trips you up in the middle of a workout, especially when you have been working hard. You'll be tempted to stop a minute and catch your breath. Before you give in to the urge, try a change of pace. Shorten your stride and speed up just slightly. Or slow down a little and push off your toes to put some bounce in your step. A change of rhythm breaks monotony and gets you in a new groove. Even a shuffle is better than a stop when it comes to mental athletics. It keeps you moving forward toward physical, mental, and spiritual fitness.

*Log In:* If you haven't started a walker's log, give it a try now. Chapter 4 suggests basic information to record. Use the log to notice patterns in your walking practice. If you miss a workout, write down the cause. Perhaps you'll see how you sabotage exercise commitments or maybe you'll discover patterns you can avoid.

Personalize your log with items that reward or motivate you. Keep track of pennies or miracles you find on your path. Record your mood or an affirmation you created. Identify a blessing you received. Your entries are markers on a spirited path. They map a route to moments of enchantment, a personalized guide to walking "in the zone" of connection with self and spirit.

*The Feeling's Mutual:* Find someone who shares your commitment to walking. Seek out a friend, a neighbor, or a work colleague who wants to develop a strong walking program. You might walk together once a week and use that opportunity to time your walking pace or experiment with walking intervals that boost your effort. It's much easier to push yourself when you feel the support of someone beside you doing the same thing.

If you walk with a companion more than once a week, make a pact to walk in silence for twenty minutes of each walk. Share energy, not social conversation or business talk. Give yourself opportunities to experience the power of supportive silence.

*Going to the Dogs:* In her book *Real Moments,* psychologist Barbara De Angelis credits her dog Bijou with guiding her into a practice of walking meditation. Rather than allowing her mind to fill with tasks and schedules, she anchors her attention on Bijou and on being "right here, right now." As she walks, she uses that phrase to stay present. "Right now, I am walking Bijou up the hill . . . right now, I am taking a deep breath of summer air . . . right now, I am looking up at the blue sky."[11]

For spirited walkers, however, dogs are more likely to provide interruption than inspiration. Workouts that strengthen both body and soul require a sustained physical effort that raises the heart rate and brings aerobic benefits. Only dogs that are well trained and physically fit enough to keep up an aerobic pace for at least twenty minutes make good workout partners for spirited walkers.

*Pick a Card:* Sometimes all you need is a gentle nudge, a nugget of daily wisdom or inspiration to give fresh meaning to your steps. Select a thought for the day from a deck of inspirational cards or affirmations and let it guide your focus on the walk. You'll find an ever-expanding selection of these specialty decks in bookstores and gift shops. Some come with angels bearing messages. Others provide an animal guide. Some give a verse of scripture for the day. Some deliver affirmations for health, prosperity, or self-acceptance.

If you enjoy pondering the mysteries of oracles or simply welcome the synchronicity of random selection in picking a thought for the day, you may find that the luck of the draw brings inspiration and fills your walks with delight and discovery.

*Just Be Cause:* Community walkathons and fund-raisers give walkers an opportunity to help others while helping themselves. When your enthusiasm for walking needs a helping hand, watch the newspapers or ask at health clubs for the dates of upcoming local events. The energy that comes from participating with a crowd in support of a good cause lasts long after the event, helping you stay in step with your own fitness goals. Recruit a group of friends to join you in the walk. If the course seems too long for one individual, make it a team effort with each walker covering a section of the route. During the walk, find someone who is walking just slightly faster than you and try to keep up. Imagine that you are attached to him or her by a cord, and let that person's energy pull you forward. Look for walkers who seem graceful and strong. Try to copy their form.

# *Side**Lines*

## TARGETING CALORIES

Weight control motivates a lot of fitness walkers to stick with a workout program. Often the steps that lead to weight loss set in motion lifestyle changes that outweigh the movement shown on the scales. If one of your goals is to lose fat and reduce body weight, the American College of Sports Medicine recommends that you exercise three to five times a week and burn at least 300 calories per session.[12] For the average walker, 300 calories means about three miles of walking.

Of course, precise calorie use varies from person to person, depending on weight, fitness, and walking speed. But if you can live with estimates and are willing to simplify the calculations, you can round off the count at 100 calories per mile and come up with an easy average.[13] Walk briskly, and you'll burn more calories per minute because you'll be covering more distance. Go uphill and you work harder, but probably move more slowly. At the end of a month, it will all even out. Consistency is what counts most when you get to the scales.

Walkers report that positive weight loss and maintenance seem to require a minimum of twelve to fifteen miles of walking per week.[14] When you exercise at a pace that puts you into your target heart range, you burn calories faster and increase cardiovascular benefits. Look at the target heart rate chart in chapter 2 to confirm your target range. As you walk, check your pulse regularly to establish a pace that is safe and effective for your goals. For general health and well-being, you probably don't need to exceed a heart rate of 50 to 60 percent of maximum heart rate. For increased fitness or weight loss, push your pulse into the 60 to 75 percent range.

Some research suggests that your exercising heart rate provides a reliable measure of calorie consumption. Exercise physiologist E. C. Frederick determined that a person with a heart rate of 120 beats per minute will burn about 10 calories a minute.[15] Sustain that heart rate for 10 minutes and you'll burn 100 calories, he says.

But keep in mind that calculations of calorie use are estimates only. Let the numbers motivate you and remember that your most reliable measure of calorie consumption may well be your waistband.

*Score a Goal:* Exercisers who achieve goals experience exhilaration and sustained motivation. Regardless of whether you set your sights on walking a mile or a marathon, you boost your chances of success when you declare a goal and work steadily toward it. Goals that encourage slow, incremental steps will keep you moving forward until your walking practice becomes integrated into daily life, as vital to well-being as brushing your teeth or eating regularly. Record goals in your walking log. Writing them down helps you get clear. Is your goal to establish a pattern of walking meditation, to lose weight, to get more fit, to have time alone, to clear your head? Focus on one aspect at a time so that you feel challenged rather than overwhelmed. Behavioral scientists from Pavlov to Skinner have recorded the natural tendency of human beings to seek immediate pleasure and avoid immediate pain. Unwieldy goals create the emotional pain of failure. Set yourself up to experience pleasure with small, achievable goals that reinforce your fitness program by providing immediate successes.

*Watch Your Language:* Pay attention to the way you talk about walking. Do you tell friends you are "trying" to walk regularly? Do you preface every reference to walking with "just"? Listen to the difference a word makes:

*For exercise, I walk.* (For exercise, I just walk.)

*I walk two miles a day.* (I just walk two miles a day.)

The same distinction occurs when you identify yourself as a walker:

*I am a walker.* (I take walks.)

By calling yourself a "walker," you make walking part of your identity. The change is very empowering. It's not something you have to "try" to become. When you change the way you talk, you begin to change the way you act. Identify yourself as a "walker," and it becomes easier to get out and walk regularly.

*Create Community:* Community colleges, health clubs, and city recreation programs all provide walking programs. Some emphasize companionship more than fitness walking, but if you ask around, you can probably locate a group of walkers who share your goals for aerobic exercise. Regular contact with other enthusiastic walkers helps renew your own commitment to a walking practice. It's also a way to pick up tips on training techniques and walking gear and to identify resources who can answer questions about fitness or shoes. If your muscles and mind are ready for advanced walking, find a racewalking class. You'll get great workouts and an opportunity to learn specialized walking techniques to practice in daily walks.

The American Volksport Association can introduce you to the pleasures of planned walks through city neighborhoods and scenic parks in the company of other dedicated walkers. The organization sponsors low-key, noncompetitive ten-kilometer walks around the country. Individuals and families of all ages and walking speeds are welcome.

The value of group participation goes beyond training tips and new trails. Community is a vital aspect of many spiritual practices. Religious orders, monastic retreats, church worship services, twelve-step groups, and weekly meditation circles all exist because they assist us to stay on the path. They support us in remembering the values and practices that provide a supporting core at the center of our lives.

# From Sole to Soul . . .

*Musical Intervals:* Poets and mystics assure us that music has the power to charm wild beasts and deadly snakes. With such strength, it's no surprise that a simple tune can turn aside the mental monsters that lurk in the shadows of our minds. This interval workout demonstrates the magic of music to subdue resistance and lead you forward to focus and fitness. Interval workouts can be done anywhere, but they provide a good excuse to head to a track where distances are easy to measure. If that's inconvenient, you can do this exercise just as successfully on a sidewalk or bike path, using a watch to measure intervals.

Allow thirty minutes for this exercise. Take five to ten minutes to warm up with easy walking. Loosen shoulders, hips, and ankles with a few gentle rotations before beginning the interval work. If you are on a track, get into position at the starting line and turn on your mental stereo. Let the simple lyrics and the crisp, clear rhythms of "Yankee Doodle Dandy" fill your mind.

With the music setting a beat, start walking fast and hard for half a lap around the track. Pump your arms and breathe into your belly. You should feel the effort. When you are halfway around the track, slow to a moderate pace and let your breathing recover as you complete the lap. When you reach the starting line again, turn up the music and pick up the momentum for another segment of fast walking. If you start receiving mental static on the way, bring your attention back to "Yankee Doodle Dandy." Sing it loudly in your mind to block out interference. At the end of half a lap, slow the pace and continue walking to the finish.

Repeat for a total of four laps, rotating fast and moderate segments without stopping for a break. The workout looks like this:

One-half lap FAST followed by one-half lap MODERATE. Repeat four times.

Do more laps if you feel ready for additional work. Take a cooldown lap around the track to let your heart rate drop gradually and gracefully at the end of your workout.

To do this exercise on a bike path or sidewalk, use an interval rotation of two minutes, alternating two minutes of fast walking with two minutes at a slightly slower pace. Repeat the rotation four times. Rely on "Yankee Doodle Dandy" to lead you safely through the temptation to slow down before you complete the two-minute burst of extra effort.

Interval workouts build fitness in a safe, gradual way. After each period of increased exertion, a short recovery phase allows you to monitor physical reactions. Did you push too hard? Not hard enough? Do you need to stop a minute and stretch your shins? Were you gasping for breath at the end? If so, should you modify your effort, or did you simply forget to breathe deep into the belly? Try breathing in rhythm with the song on the next segment.

Once you've learned to sing yourself past resistance, you will have mastered a fitness technique you can take with you anywhere, anytime, to calm the beasts in your mind. Expand your repertoire of songs with personal favorites or rousing standards such as "I've Been Working on the Railroad."

*Pick Up the Beat:* Variety is essential to motivation. If you begin to tire of your own voice and want someone else to entertain you, let programmed walking tapes orchestrate your walks occasionally. Fitness walking tapes that keep you moving at a consistent speed throughout a workout are available at paces to suit walkers of all levels. This exercise determines what pace is appropriate for you. It also provides a challenge in mental athletics.

You'll need a sports watch with numbers that are easy to read for this exercise. It may be helpful to wear the watch with the dial on the inside of your wrist, enabling you to see the face without effort when your arm swings forward. You'll time yourself for one minute as you count your steps.

Make sure that you are thoroughly warmed up before starting the exercise. Build speed gradually until you reach a pace that pushes you just beyond the comfort zone. You want a speed that gives you an aerobic workout—increased heart rate and breathing level—without forcing you to a level of exertion that creates risk.

Once you've reached your aerobic pace, get ready to time yourself. All you have to do is count your steps while maintaining the pace for one minute. Focus your attention on one foot only, counting each time that foot hits the ground. At the end of a minute, double the number to give

you the total number of steps per minute. Check yourself
by repeating the one-minute count several times. This is
more than a test of accuracy; it's also an exercise in focused
awareness. You'll discover that even one minute can be too
long to hold the awareness steady. Something will distract
you. Your attention will wander and you'll falter on the
numbers. You'll forget which foot you're counting. Nothing
to do when this happens except to begin anew, as in the
practice of meditation. Draw your focus back to your steps.

You'll probably find that your one-minute count falls
somewhere between 110 and 170 steps. Specialty walking
tapes are programmed to maintain a certain walking speed
or to provide a specific number of footsteps, or beats, per
minute. Sports stores and fitness catalogs carry walking
tapes with a steady beat. Select a speed that matches your
aerobic pace. Choose a tape of instrumental music without
lyrics so you can focus on mental imagery while picking up
the beat. The resource section at the back of this book
includes source information.

*Silent Centipede:* This exercise invites you to reconnect with
the joys of Follow the Leader, giving you an opportunity to
feel the physical and emotional delight that emerge when
you move in smooth harmony with another person. You
may be two people or a group of several. Numbers and
speed don't matter here; mindfulness is the goal.

Try this experiment on a track or on a jogging trail
where you won't feel conspicuous when you drop into
centipede formation. Allow thirty minutes for the exercise.

Begin with a warm-up walk of five to ten minutes. Loosen ankles, waist, shoulders, and hips with a few easy rotations. Stretch the shins if you feel tightness in the front of the legs.

While loosening up, decide how long each person will hold the lead. One lap around a track is a good distance. Or one quarter of a mile on a bike trail. If possible, each segment should be at least three minutes long so that followers have time to feel the rhythm of moving in rapport.

Line up single file behind the leader, giving the leader plenty of space to set the pace without feeling pushed. As the line begins to move, place your full attention on the person immediately in front of you. Be mindful of arm swing, pace, and stride length as you attempt to duplicate these movements with your own body.

When it is time to rotate the lead, the first person simply steps aside in silence and drops to the end of the line. The second person becomes the leader, free to set a different pace and speed, without speaking or explaining the changes. Repeat the rotation in periods of three to five minutes for a silent workout of at least twenty minutes.

As a variation, you might use this centipede formation for an exercise that builds intensity and speed gradually. Starting slowly, let the pace increase with each change of leadership. With the support of group energy, you will probably notice that you are able to walk faster and sustain the pace longer than you can alone.

One of the benefits of spirited walking is the period of retreat that it creates in the midst of busy lives. When you walk with friends in silence, you expand the retreat as you learn to communicate with movement and mindfulness rather than with words. If you usually talk business with colleagues or visit with friends while you walk, you may not be comfortable with silence at first. Be patient. With practice you will discover the pure support that silence can convey.

# CHAPTER 8

~

# A Healing Path

## TAKING STRIFE IN STRIDE

In the evening, when the Phoenix sun dipped behind the horizon and the air began to cool, Stephanie Deer emerged like a shadow to walk the dry channel of a desert wash. As she walked, she'd fill her lungs with air, unconscious of the fragrance that hung in the warmth of dusk. She thought only of release—of letting go of the pain clamped inside. With each exhalation she loosed a sigh. In and out. Breathe and sigh. The cycle built slowly until sighs billowed into moans and then emerged as roars.

As the darkness deepened along her path, the tears began to flow. Night after night, she walked the riverbed, splashing it with the grief and anger that followed her husband's suicide. "It was my cleansing, my healing," she says. "I could walk that wash and just cry."[1]

During the day, she struggled to maintain balance in the unfamiliar roles and responsibilities hurled on her by his desperate act. Panic attacks shook her so fiercely that she pulled her car to the side of the road and vomited on the way to meetings with her husband's former business associates. "Suicide—that kind of shock doesn't ever go away, but I learned that I was a really strong person and that I could cope. Walking helped me do that. I don't know what I would do if I couldn't walk," she says.

Six years after her husband's death, Stephanie walks five times a week, usually for an hour. Sometimes she walks with a friend, but often she spends the time alone. She calls it her hour with God. "My feet hit the ground and I say, 'Thank you, God, for this day.' Then I try not to think anything. What's important is that I do the breathing that lets me mentally or emotionally cleanse. Walking has had a tremendous effect on my recovery."

Increasingly, research is confirming what walkers like Stephanie already know: in times of crisis and stress, walking leads to healing paths. Simply finding the strength to put one foot in front of the other invokes an innate will to survive. When depression and grief numb the body, walking awakens the profound healing powers of the human spirit.

From bad moods to broken hearts, the emotional benefits of walking seem almost as indisputable as its contributions to physical health. At Duke University, researchers determined that exercise is as effective as medication in reducing symptoms of depression.[2] At California State University, research psychologist Robert E. Thayer demonstrated that even ten minutes of energetic walking can lift a person's spirits. After probing the relationship of exercise and mental state, Thayer reports that exercise is the best prescription for the blahs or a bad mood.[3] Scientists say that's because exercise sets in motion chemical changes that bring new vitality to the cells. Walking releases chemicals in the brain that literally change the way we feel. At the same time, it burns stress-producing hormones that build up when the body is inactive.

Most people feel the benefits of a ten-minute walk for an hour or more afterward. Longer walks bring longer-lasting results, but don't let a lack of time stall you. Even five minutes of walking can reduce anxiety and improve attitude. And repetition doesn't dull the impact. The positive influence on energy, mood, and self-esteem occurs every time you exercise—day after day after day.

All of this biochemical wizardry was taken for granted by people such as my grandfather who worked a small farm in the Oregon hills and herded his milk cows into the barn each night on foot. Only in recent years have we created industrial cultures in which exercise must be intentionally added to our lifestyles. Cars, elevators, television, and drive-up windows have made us increasingly sedentary, distancing us from the natural healing powers our bodies release with activity.

Unfortunately, the times when we most need something to alter mood or energy are often the times when we feel unable to move. Grief and depression can immobilize the muscles, creating a fatigue that weighs the body down. Although nothing prepares one for life's jolts, we may survive times of stress better if regular exercise is an established pattern in our lives. Habits sustain us when we can't think clearly. A person who has experienced the benefits of daily walks may find it easier to muster what Thayer calls "cognitive override"—the ability to grit your teeth and do what you know is best. Pace the floor, walk up and down a hallway, stroll around the block—even if you really don't feel like it. In moving, you take a step toward positive change.

## WORKING OUT AND WORKING THROUGH

Before Madeline Hersh took her first steps, her parents pushed her stroller along New York City sidewalks for Sunday outings to Brighton Beach, three miles from their home. They held her hand when she grew strong enough to toddle beside them on the route. In her carless urban family, walking was a well-established tradition.

The tradition continued when Madeline married and walked with children of her own. Then, when life handed her a one-two-three punch of tragedies in a single year, walking led her through a dense fog of despair. The first blow came when a rapid form of cancer claimed the life of her beloved father. Two months later, another foundation gave way when she lost her job as a graphic artist. Before she recovered from that shock, the company that had employed her husband for thirty-two years shut down, leaving both of them unemployed.

"In the beginning I walked to escape when the walls closed in," she says.[4] "It was almost a fanatical need to keep going. I realize now that I was looking for some place to put my feet that didn't give way under me. When everything looked hopeless, I walked through it."

Some days, she walked the streets of her suburban New Jersey neighborhood until her legs and back ached. In the stillness of the house, her husband grieved his own loss. Madeline concealed her pain until it pressed against her throat in waves of nausea. Then she pulled the door shut behind her and felt the earth beneath her feet again. She walked through nausea and through tears until she reached a sense of clarity.

"When I felt myself getting depressed and feeling the world was going to crush me, I put on my sneakers and went out to walk. When I didn't want to go, I went anyway. For me, it was fighting back the demons. All of a sudden, nothing was working the way it was supposed to, and nothing I did could change what was happening. The only thing I could control was what I did with myself."

For eighteen months, she paced the streets in search of stability. She often walked three or four times a day. At night she wore a reflective vest. In winter, she fell into step behind the snowplow. "Months later, I realized that going out to walk was the way I was healing. It's like I walked into a new life."

Madeline's new life led to a stimulating position as a public information officer and television show host. But it didn't change her relationship with walking. Morning walks allow her to prepare for the day ahead. Evening outings with a daughter who lives nearby carry on a family tradition. She counts on one hand the number of days of walking she has missed in the three years since her father's death. What keeps her going is the clarity that comes when feet and heart and lungs work together to create a rhythm.

"There is a peace that comes, and my mind relaxes. This is my spirituality—my connection to God, if you will, or to keeping in touch with who I am. This is what I do for myself. It's my most peaceful time and it has always worked for me. That's where the clarity comes in."

## IN STEP WITH HEALING

The integration of mind and body for healing has a rich heritage in human history. Long before today's medical experts concluded that a brisk walk is a step in the right direction, the ancient Greek physician Hippocrates prescribed morning and evening walks for a variety of illnesses. Honored as the father of modern medicine, Hippocrates advocated fresh air, exercise, and proper diet more than two thousand years ago.[5]

After centuries of medical specialization and scientific isolation, contemporary medical authorities are circling back to Hippocrates' commonsense prescription for healthy living. The U.S. surgeon general advocates a holistic approach to health and wellness that could have come from ancient Greece: to expand the length and quality of your life, make physical fitness a daily habit. The recommendation rests on clear evidence that exercise builds strong bodies and strong spirits.

The physical benefits of walking are sufficient to produce significant biological and emotional changes, but spirited walking can magnify the healing power of a brisk step. Spirited walking restores the mental and physical connection that is often severed by fear and tragedy. When walkers accompany their steps with healing words and images, they carry a candle of illumination that guides their passage through the labyrinth of despair.

Psychologists say that when we feel blue, our minds turn into broken records. Our thoughts loop endlessly over the same laments: *I can't do this. I'm afraid. I feel tired. I'll never finish. I'm not good enough.* Harvard physician Herbert Benson warns that when we "marinate our minds in negativity and fear," we trigger the body's flight-or-fight response and lock our systems in an ever-deepening spiral of worry. Benson's landmark research into the health benefits of meditation identified a mental state he calls the "relaxation response," in which the body relaxes and restores itself. Repetition of a word, a phrase, or a pattern of movement such as walking interrupts the loop of mental worry and guides the body into the "relaxation response."

When a relaxed physical state is combined with positive mental messages such as affirmations and prayers, Benson believes that it is possible to "rewire" the body's automatic responses to stress. He calls the process "cognitive restructuring"—literally, an opportunity to change your mind by replacing negative self-talk with positive messages of strength and faith.[6]

Some mental-health professionals acknowledge the healing power of movement by inviting clients to put on walking shoes and step outside. Therapists who offer counseling sessions on foot maintain that walking relaxes people, making it easier to talk about stressful situations. In addition to walking during sessions, they are likely to prescribe several healthy walks a week for willing clients. But even without the assistance of a therapist, spirited walking often leads to emotional healing. Spirited walking interrupts automatic responses to stress. It stops the flow of negative self-talk and pulls awareness into the present. Affirmations, mantras, poems, and prayers become internal "therapists" redirecting the focus to thoughts that provide inspiration and reassurance.

Many people find that words of poetry or scripture calm the storms that buffet us in times of emotional stress. Advocates of poetry therapy blend psychology and literature in the treatment of stress. Simply repeating meaningful lines of poetry while walking can reduce anxiety, they say.[7] Poetry lets us know that we are not alone. By identifying feelings or beliefs we hold, poems assure us that someone else understands what we are experiencing. Poems validate our grief, our joy, our sorrow, our loneliness. In reciting them, we make a conscious choice to seek a larger view, to take refuge from the storm in a moment of retreat, accompanied by poets, mystics, or the divine guidance of a higher power.

If you have a favorite poem or prayer, don't wait until your world is crumbling to call on it for emotional support. Memorize two or three passages that offer inspiration, sending a beacon of connection and belonging through your daily walks. Look for verses, phrases, or affirmations that give you strength in times of difficulty and delight in times of ease. Make them familiar companions on your walks.

If you don't have a favorite, Linus Mundy, author of *Prayer-Walking*, suggests the Lord's Prayer or "Not my will but thine" as starting places for walkers who want to strengthen awareness of God's presence. "Realize, as you walk, that your real journey is an interior one. You are looking for love and opening up to Grace," he says.[8]

Feel free to personalize the lines that you memorize. Change pronouns to "I" and "me" if you want to make the message more personal. Replace "God" with "higher power" or "divine mind" if you identify with a broader deity. Select words that penetrate your core. Hear them with the soul. Imagine starting each walk with a soaring invocation like these lines from the poet Eugene Guillevic:

> *When each day*
> *is sacred*
>
> *when each hour*
> *is sacred*
>
> *when each instant*
> *is sacred*
>
> *earth and you*
> *space and you*
> *bearing the sacred*
> *through time*
>
> *you'll reach*
> *the fields of light.*[9]

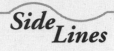

## POETRY IN MOTION

When the body moves, we physically change position and perspective. If that action is echoed by movement in the mind, we initiate changes in thoughts and emotions as well. Poetry, prayers, and blessings focus that mental movement on words that heal. They guide us toward connection with ourselves, with nature, with humanity, and with the beliefs that support and sustain us. When you memorize a poem or a spiritually inspiring passage, you commit the words to heart. Walking carries them throughout the body.

When you repeat a poem or passage daily as part of a walking practice, the pattern establishes a ritual that gives meaning to each day. Repetition creates reassurance that some things in life remain constant. The words ignite a comforting glow that warms the soul like the voice of a friend. They guide the feet through detours on life's path.

Experiment with poems in this chapter, or select other passages that have special meaning for you. Jot down the words on a three-by-five index card and carry it while you walk until you memorize the lines.

*Happily may I walk.*
*Happily, with abundant dark clouds, may I walk.*
*Happily, with abundant showers, may I walk.*
*Happily, with abundant plants, may I walk.*
*Happily, on a trail of pollen, may I walk.*
*Happily may I walk.*
*Being as it used to be long ago, may I walk.*

NAVAJO CHANT[10]

*Help us to be the always hopeful*
*Gardeners of the spirit*
*Who know that without darkness*
*Nothing comes to birth*
*As without light*
*Nothing flowers.*

MAY SARTON[11]

*That is perfect.*
*This is perfect.*
*Perfect comes from perfect.*
*Take perfect from perfect,*
*the remainder is perfect.*
*May peace and peace and peace be everywhere.*

THE UPANISHADS[12]

*And yet, there is only*
*One great thing,*
*The only thing:*
*To live to see in huts and on journeys*
*The great day that dawns,*
*And the light that fills the world.*

INUIT SONG[13]

Mystics through the ages have written about the spark of light that illuminates the soul. Its glow, they say, reveals the divinity within us—the godliness that glows at the core of every being. To discover this light and to walk in its brilliance are life's highest goals. With Guillevic's words as a guide, daily workouts become paths of spiritual discovery that can lead us occasionally into "fields of light" where every step is sacred.

## A PATH TO CREATIVE RECOVERY

The healing power of walking reveals itself most dramatically in times of emotional crisis, but it can also ease the everyday slumps that send us to the vending machine in the middle of the afternoon for a bar of energy. It can smooth out deadlines, delays, and disagreements. Leadership development consultant Kay Gilley considers short walking breaks an ideal prescription for boosting work productivity and stimulating creative breakthroughs.[14]

Gilley discovered the restorative powers of walking when a freak jogging accident flipped her life off course. An avid runner, she tripped one morning in the rain and injured a spinal disk. The fall detoured her into a rehabilitation program where she spent two years learning to dress herself, and then to walk. An arduous recovery taught her to value each step as a meditation. Movement came only when she held her focus firmly in the present, forging a cooperative effort of muscles and mind.

Eight years after the accident, she runs again for exercise, but she walks when she gets stuck. The process that guided her to physical healing now smoothes her passage through the mental challenges she encounters as an author and consultant. "There is something about backing off and getting into a relaxed space that I think lets us access a spiritual part of ourselves," she says. "What is important is to get your mind off the problem and take yourself into a bigger space of the collective unconscious, or the universal global brain— whatever you want to call it."

While working on *The Alchemy of Fear*, a guide to spiritual awareness in the workplace, Gilley took frequent walks. "Usually within twenty to forty minutes I would have an answer. Sometimes I didn't understand exactly what it meant until I started writing, but it was always an important piece."

Miles of pathways weave through the North Carolina woods near her home, providing a rich setting for connection with internal and external inspiration. But creative problem solving can occur anywhere. In a parking lot or on a treadmill, the repetitious rhythm of aerobic walking can trigger corresponding movement in mental clarity, emotions, and energy. It can open the mind to its own internal wisdom. The secret to gaining access to that wisdom lies in learning to still the voices that assail us when we feel uncertain and insecure. As Gilley walks, she avoids thinking about problems. Sometimes she fixes attention on one foot, feeling each part of its movement through a step. Sometimes she focuses on the swing of her arms. Anything to free her mind from the repetitious thought cycles that lead to creative dead ends.

Focusing tools provide a break from mental chatter. They offer a healing respite from frustration, grief, or fear.

But focus demands practice and persistence. The sense of peace it offers comes only when we learn to make the conscious choice to step aside for a moment, out of the eddy of "what if" and "why me" that spins us off course. Rarely does one escape the swirl without effort.

When I left a longtime position as a newspaper reporter, it seemed enormously important to me that I demonstrate quickly my ability to succeed as an independent writer. My ego lusted after bylines in glossy periodicals as evidence that I had made no mistake in leaving a secure position. It wanted special assignments and impressive credentials to roll out when friends and former colleagues asked, "What are you doing these days?"

*Newsweek*'s decision to publish a personal opinion essay that I submitted sent my aspirations soaring.[15] Then came a painful trail of rejections. Weeks stretched into months of byline anonymity. One overcast February day, the fax machine spewed out a rejection letter from the editor of a prestigious magazine and my resilience snapped. I slumped at my desk and felt a tsunami of doubt crash against my heart. Twice I had revised the article in response to his suggestions. That's nice, he had said, after the first change, but he wondered if perhaps I could expand it. Then it would be just right. Now I stared at the fax and saw only failure in the courtesies of "not for us, after all . . . please think of us in the future."

The words uncaged a waiting terror. I headed out the door, hoping to outwalk the fear of failure that snapped at my heels like a surly street cur. I felt its presence at my back and heard the threats rattling in its throat: *Get a job,* it taunted. *Just go get a job. Get a job. Give it up. Get a job.*

As rain streaked my glasses, I tried to dodge the words by walking faster. I grasped at mental diversions. I counted steps. I snatched at mantras and walked through a downpour of confusion. *One, two, three, four . . . Get a job, get a job . . . I am here and I am clear . . . Get a job, go get a job.* Urgently, I scrambled for words I could cling to. *I am clear, com-pas-sion-ate, and liv-ing in my power,* I chanted, hoping the phrase would restore my balance.

Over and over, fears assailed me. With practiced stealthiness, they slipped beneath the surface of my concentration and chanted in the background of my mind like the pulse of an hypnotic drum. Time and again, I shook the fear-trance from my head. *I am here and I am clear.* The affirmation guided the rhythm of my steps, creating a spirited pace that silenced the drumbeat for a moment.

Thirty minutes out, I passed the soccer field and headed toward home. My body had settled into a soothing rhythm and the storm inside seemed to be subsiding. I gave thanks for health and for the strength to keep moving, maintaining my stride in turbulent times. In that instant, I tripped again. *Maybe this isn't what I should be doing with my life. Maybe I'm not listening to guidance.* A crippling uncertainty hobbled my steps.

*Not now,* I pleaded. *Not now, please. No more problem solving now.* Once again I returned to affirmations, seeking to reach with words and muscles the sense of balance that rests on a sustaining faith that the spirit within me is clear and strong. The words carried me home to try once more—aching, yes, bruised from a tumble, but steady enough to take another step.

Like physical balance, spiritual and emotional balance do not occur automatically for most of us. Balance rewards a willingness to step forward in thin air, to teeter in uncertainty and risk a spill. Children grasp for helping hands and table legs while they practice the physical balance that eventually enables them to stand on their own. First steps are awkward; they bring repeated failure and the pain of bumped heads. Still, children try to stand again.

Language reflects the way that grief and emotional pain return us to the instability of toddlers. Bad news "kicks our legs out from under us." Difficulties "throw us off stride" and "knock the wind out of us." Like the disastrous fall that forced Kay Gilley to relearn the balance of walking, emotional falls hurl us back to the basics of conscious choice. Gilley didn't ask herself if the accident was a sign that she should give up walking. She made a choice to start again. This time her steps led to spiritual alchemy, a transformation that turns setbacks into blessings. "This injury got me into touch with my spirit, which I had ignored for years," she says.

Spirited walking expands the mental and physical support available to us when we feel off balance. Each time we make an intentional choice to try again, we strengthen the rhythms that lead body and mind into balance. Each time we reach for the support of our own breath, or for the stability of a reassuring passage, we reconnect with the truths that hold us upright. In those moments of contact, we touch the outstretched hand of a higher power. Call it inner wisdom or divine guidance, it steadies us until we find the courage to take another step.

Each time that mind and body align with a clear focus, the union echoes through cells and synapses, opening new channels of physical and spiritual communication. Those moments flood the soul with reminders that "when each day is sacred . . . when each instant is sacred . . . you'll reach the fields of light."

# From Sole to Soul . . .

*On Solid Ground:* "Keep your feet on the ground," we tell ourselves in moments of stress or confusion. When we need clarity, we know the importance of staying firmly rooted in the present rather than allowing fear or stress to send us soaring into thin air.

"Keep your feet on the ground" is good advice both mentally and physically. It brings us in contact with a solid base of support. Walking restores that connection when emotions send us spinning. To increase your awareness of the stable earth beneath your feet, try this experiment for a few minutes during a workout or hike. You'll want a smooth, level surface that provides solid footing. Take time to warm up thoroughly and loosen the ankles with some foot rotations before starting. Focus on mental awareness rather than walking speed at first.

Begin by imitating a tin soldier's stiff-kneed strut for a minute or two. Lift your toes in the air and land on the heels. Your movements will feel rigid and jerky as you march forward like a toy.

Now contrast the awkwardness of tin-soldier struts by imagining that each foot is a rocker on a comfortable rocking chair. With each step, roll the full length of each rocker. Notice your heel contacting the ground below your body. Feel your weight roll forward across the arch and lift gently onto the ball of the foot. Finish each step with a push off from the toes. Roll forward smoothly, using the strength and power in the entire foot.

By rolling forward through the toes, you move in a pattern that literally "keeps your feet on the ground" a little longer and prolongs connection with a supportive earth. You'll also be learning a walking technique that boosts speed and turnover rate by giving each step a send-off.

*Take a Breather:* When tension grips the body, it is very common for breathing to become shallow and irregular. Therapists say that people in pain and stress have a tendency to take a deep breath and hold it, as if trying to hold back their fears. By holding the breath, we heighten anxiety and lock fear inside the body. This exercise gives the body a good airing out, releasing the mental and chemical toxins that inhibit well-being.

As you begin the warm-up phase of your walk, become aware of your breath. Allow a deep rhythmic pattern of breathing to develop, and simply be mindful of the pattern for a few minutes. When your body has settled into a comfortable rhythm of moving and breathing, check your watch or set the timer for five minutes. Begin to count your footsteps as you inhale and exhale. Try to stretch the breath out for three or four steps on each in and out. Pull the breath into the belly so you feel your diaphragm expand. Release the air in a steady flow. Continue the counting until five minutes is up. When your mind strays, bring your attention back to the count. Think of nothing except counting the steps with each breath.

At the end of five minutes, set your timer for five minutes more. This time, instead of counting, add visual images or words to each breath so that you create an active flow of energy in and out of the body. Imagine that each breath fills your cells with new life. Let each exhalation remove anything that blocks the energy. Pretend, for example, that the air you inhale carries rich, red fuel from the earth below you. Let its vibrant life fill your cells with renewal. Notice its movement through your legs and feel it roll across the tension in the shoulders. Exhale out the top of your head, releasing anger, resentment, grief, or muscle tightness into the sky. Imagine it floating away, creating space in the body for fresh air and new growth.

Alternate the two breathing exercises in five-minute segments to give yourself at least twenty minutes of conscious breathing. Increase walking speed gradually during the workout so that your breathing becomes aerobic and full as the body makes room for more air. People who exercise regularly and aerobically literally create more capillary space, increasing their capacity to nourish and cleanse the body's internal systems.

# CHAPTER 9

~

## *Peak Experiences*
### On a Trail of Discovery

Heavy rains dumped a sullen mood on the string of hikers plodding along a mountain trail in Nepal. For three days, we had trudged in damp discomfort beneath steamy rain gear and a soggy sky. Drops of water spilled from the polished leaves of rhododendron bushes along the path. Wiry black tendrils undulated on the limbs of shrubs that drooped into the trail. Leeches. Tentacles of horror arcing into the air in search of flesh. Our clothing wore signs of their success in the blood-red badges that stained socks and sleeves.

By now, the rain had permeated the black cotton umbrella I purchased in Kathmandu at the beginning of this twenty-day trek in the Himalayan highlands. I held its sodden weight above my head and smoldered beneath its dark cover. Clouds obscured the world's highest peaks. The umbrella confined my view to a tight circle at my feet. In its circumference I saw only mud and leeches and burning money. My money. Savings that I had decided to risk on adventure. I huddled under a canopy of self-criticism and told myself that I'd been foolish.

As a novice hiker, I was unprepared for the mental challenges of this journey. It came less than a year after my initiation to serious hiking in the mountains of Arizona. But the travel brochure had promised Hindu shrines and Buddhist monasteries. It offered meetings with spiritual teachers. I imagined a hike of divine inspiration. Leeches and mud and musty clothing never entered my thoughts.

Now my mind howled in outrage: *Why did I come here? How long can this go on? How fast can I get out?* The questions pummeled my brain. The nearest road lay three or four days behind at Jiri where we had started walking. The airport at Lukla was almost the same distance ahead. Stuck in the middle, cut off from past and future, there was little to do but keep moving.

Slowly, a sort of numbness encompassed me. Incantations of rage gave way to prayer as my mind retreated into monotony. The rain had outlasted me. *"Om mani padme hum,"* I mumbled mechanically, adopting as a mantra the Sanskrit words carved in stone at every turn on these distant trails. The ancient blessing pays homage to the spark of divinity that burns in the heart of every living thing. Sherpa guides walk with the phrase on their lips. Village women drone it ceaselessly. Chanting it diluted my frustration at traveling around the world for mountains I could not see. By the time the clouds rose from Everest, Lhotse, and Ama Dablam, my attitude and my vision had improved. The broad umbrella above my head had assumed the shape of a spiritual tool.

Inexplicably, the space beneath the black canopy expanded as I settled into a rhythm of steps and words. Within its confines, I found a sanctuary—a meditative retreat into mindfulness, a peaceful cloister constructed from the present moment. Inside its shelter, I walked with mystics and rinpoches, letting my body integrate words that had simply slid through me before. Acceptance seeped into my cells, silent and unseen. For delicate fragments of time, past and future fell away, and I hung suspended in the present, moving forward one step at a time—seeking the spark of divinity in everything.

My path along the mud-slick trails of Nepal reached a destination not described in the brochure. It led me past wind-whipped prayer flags atop a 13,000-foot pass and carried me into villages where the cymbals and horns of Buddhist monasteries roused me from sleep with a spiritual chaos that spilled into the dawn like laughter. But more important, the route delivered me to a fuller image of myself as a physical and spiritual being. Trekking restored a sense of awe and connection that I had lost. Hiking boots and a backpack became my vestments in a form of worship that has transformed me into a pilgrim, a postulant in a vast order of walkers who find wholeness and holiness on foot.

Hiking brings us into contact with nature and with our own divine nature. What we encounter changes us. We go to the mountain, says the poet René Daumal, not because we can stay on the summit forever but because the experience forever changes the way we live when we return to the valley. "One climbs, one sees. One descends, one sees no longer but has seen. There is an art of conducting oneself in the lower regions by the memory of what one saw higher up. When one can no longer see, one can at least still know."[1]

Encounters with nature have the power to lead us beyond our human limits, to shrink our mortal fears, concerns, and goals for a moment and restore connection with forces greater than ourselves. Nature facilitates communication with inner wisdom and higher powers, however you define them. Regardless of whether we climb the Himalayas or a gentle hill at the edge of town, we make an expedition into ourselves.

## A Trail to Spiritual Summits

For walkers, something magical happens on a hillside. When the mind relaxes and the muscles ease into a steady rhythmic movement, the spirit is free to fly. Mountain climbers often talk about "going to church" when they describe the peaks that beckon them with physical challenges and spiritual rewards. They go to the mountain as a form of worship, a connection with the strongest, highest parts of themselves. They go for the alchemy of body, mind, and spirit that transforms a physical challenge into a "peak experience."

"I am closer to God in the mountains, plain and simple," confirms climber Margo Chisholm. "Each of us has our own idea of what god is. It isn't about church. It's about the essence of what god is, a higher power. On a trail, I feel that—whether it's Everest or a trail where I can still see houses. The essence is still there. Being on a mountain is what fills me."[2]

The miracle still amazes her. Before she discovered the spiritual nourishment of mountain trails, Margo had filled the emptiness inside with sugar, alcohol, and drugs. She had a thousand-dollar-a-week cocaine habit and a serious eating disorder. She topped off Twinkies and Snickers bars with purgatives, consuming up to ninety laxatives a day and pushing her body into a chemical imbalance that nearly ended her life. At age thirty-eight, she landed in a detox program where physicians informed her that she was four months from death if she continued her patterns of abuse. Fear sent her into recovery and helped her retrieve both her health and her dreams.

Memories of her grandfather's carved elephant collection guided her to an African safari. They rekindled a dream to scale the lofty heights of Mount Kilimanjaro, the highest peak on the African continent. Step by step, she reached the summit and gained a new view of life. "One step at a time was how I learned to make it through a day in treatment," she wrote in an account of her journey. "The same simple principles worked as well on this mountain as on the ones I was climbing inside. Show up, put one foot in front of the other, and extraordinary things can happen."[3]

At the top of Kilimanjaro, Margo felt something snap open inside her. It was a box of lost ambitions: "I want to hike. I want to trek. I want to stand on the top of mountains." In a moment of exhaustion, triumph, and bitter cold, she felt a new rush of possibility and potential. Elation rose from the volcanic cinders of Kilimanjaro's 19,340-foot peak, a pinnacle named Uhuru Point—a word that means "freedom" in Swahili.[4] Out of triumph, a challenge grew: Margo embarked on a quest to become the first woman to scale the Seven Summits—the highest point on each continent.

When she had conquered six, she trained for Everest. Twice she joined climbing expeditions bound for the top of the world. Twice, the slopes of Everest defeated her, forcing her to retreat in illness. "Enough," she decided. She'd achieved a summit not plotted on contour maps. The metaphor of physical challenge, of preparing carefully and moving forward steadily, had charted a route for the rest of her life. "My Everest happened to be Everest. We all have our Everest. It doesn't have to be big, or long, or hard. It's the dream that matters," she says.

The survival skills that Margo learned from mountain summits now guide her along a safer path through daily life. Hikes on the Rocky Mountain slopes that cradle her home remind her to live one step at a time, fully present in each moment. On a trail, away from paved streets and car engines, she reconnects quickly with the immense sense of possibility that she discovered on Kilimanjaro. Even short hikes carry her to a joyous summit—a sense of gratitude and awe. "I walk half an hour up and then I come back down. I am never out of sight of civilization, but it fills my soul again." As she walks, she chats with a god who likes to hike. Sometimes she punctuates her footsteps with an empowering prayer: "God's love, God's strength, God's will, I can," she chants. The words connect her to a supportive friend who holds her when she needs a listener, a higher power who knows what's going on and can guide the course of her life.

## REFLECTIONS IN NATURE'S MIRROR

Nature leads us along trails of transformation. Spend an hour, a day, or a week hiking in nature, and we return home changed. Hiking balances body and soul. Moods improve. Creativity increases. When we free our senses from the interference of schedules, clocks, and news reports, we reconnect with the vitality and sustaining power of life. We hear and see differently. In nature's mirror we glimpse the best of ourselves.

"At some stage of every day's hiking, or almost every day's hiking, there comes a moment when your cerebral synapses seem to click into gear," observes author Colin Fletcher, whose guidebooks have introduced a generation of backpackers to the outdoors.[5] "For a few minutes or half an hour or perhaps even for the rest of the day, you fire on all cylinders. You soar, embrace the universe, see everything, solve the insoluble at a glance—you operate, that is, the way you wish you always did."

That magical moment of well-being appears on short walks as well as long ones. It requires neither discomfort nor stress. It pays no heed to endurance tests or elevation gains. It arrives in the instant that you are able to step from one world into another. As you establish a daily walking practice and discover the joy of moving from sole to soul on a path toward fitness for the whole body, hiking expands your horizons. Hiking is simply walking in nature, but it opens us to broader vistas and new perspectives that are both internal and external.

Mark Black, director of hiking at Canyon Ranch fitness spa in Arizona, has been watching hikers make the journey for fifteen years. Vacationers sign up for their first hike into the scenic wilderness near the resort because they want the exercise. They return for a second and third mountain outing because they find something more, he says. "Hiking is excellent exercise, but that's a side effect of why people come back. I think they come for the way it affects them internally—spiritually, psychologically, mentally."[6]

Hiking brings down the walls between people and nature, Mark says. It awakens a timeless rhythm that alters a walker's frame of mind. "It's like doing yoga or meditation. If you practice meditation every day, it spills over into how you perceive reality. That is the reason I studied martial arts for ten years. Hiking does the same thing. It will change your life. Whenever I go on a hike, no matter how I feel, I always know that I'll come back somehow better."

The course of Mark's life, both on and off the job, draws direction from hiking trails. Before a day in the office as coordinator of a program that takes eleven thousand hikers

# *Side**Lines*

## PRINTS OF PEACE

Walking meditation plays an important role in many spiritual practices. At meditation retreats, it provides intervals of movement between periods of sitting meditation. Sometimes walking meditation becomes an elaborate ritual in which hands, feet, and mind come together in a dance of mindfulness and prayer. Traditionally, walking meditations are done slowly, at a pace that stills the body as well as the mind.

When you've had a day filled with activity and what you need most is to quiet your mind so that you can reconnect with nature—and with your own divine nature—experiment with contemplative walking meditation. Pick a location where you can focus fully on your steps. It might be a hallway or your living room. Perhaps you know a quiet path outdoors. Lower your eyes and turn your attention to your steps. Walk slowly, counting each step in a pattern of one to four. When your attention strays, simply begin the count again. Or focus on your breathing, blocking out mental chatter by thinking "in" as you inhale and "out" as you release each breath.

Thich Nhat Hanh, Vietnamese Buddhist monk and peace activist, teaches meditation students to plant peace and happiness on the earth with each step. Instead of letting thoughts of difficulty and unhappiness course through your stride, think peace, he says. Walk in a relaxed, mindful manner. Be aware of your foot touching the ground and consciously imprint peace with each step. Think about leaving footprints that heal the earth.

195

Sorrow and fear pollute the pure soil, he says. Peace and happiness restore purity. "The pure land is in our minds. It depends on our way of making steps."[7] Walking on the earth with thoughts of peace is a way of massaging the earth with our feet, planting seeds of joy and happiness with each step.

Walking meditation is not a means to an end, he says. It *is* the end. By walking with reverence and dignity we nourish ourselves and the earth. Our steps demonstrate awareness and gratitude for the earth's gifts and for spiritual guidance. Make each step an expression of your spirit. In this way, he says, "Our Mother will heal us, and we will heal her."[8]

a year into nature, Mark frequently prepares with a hike of his own. His route carries him three miles up a rugged trail to Blackett's Ridge, a rocky promontory overlooking Sabino Canyon. At the top, he turns and clears his mind. He leans forward and lets momentum build as he descends the trail on a run. A keen fusion of muscles and mind guide him down a precipitous course between rocks and cactus spines. "We're talking thirty minutes of sustained ultra-focus," he says. "It has replaced what used to be my formal meditation. It does what meditation does, this sense of harmony and peace. You don't need to go out there and do yoga on the mountain. You just have to let the mountain do its thing."

Mountains are powerful metaphors for climbers and seekers of all kinds. They are symbols of heightened awareness, challenge, and achievement. The "mountain" you climb as a hiker might be a level trail through a river canyon or a rolling path along a grassy hillside. Every trail reveals its own challenges and rewards to those who walk it mindfully.

Community recreation centers often offer hiking opportunities that invite you to explore the outdoors in the company of knowledgeable leaders. Local outdoor clubs may sponsor weekend hikes. Check the outdoor section of the newspaper for listings, or ask at the YMCA. Hike leaders can help you select outings that are appropriate for your fitness level. "You come home a little tired, but you feel better, not only physically but mentally as well. It gives you a high—a good feeling about life," observes a Colorado hiker who shows up often on summer hikes sponsored by a local senior center.

Seek out routes that provide at least an hour or two of steady walking. Start slowly, giving your body time to warm up and find balance on irregular surfaces. Avoid the temptation to "attack" the trail by setting off at a pace that can quickly exhaust you. Pay attention to your breathing and let it guide your exertion level. Practice drawing fresh air deep into your abdomen to fuel the body with oxygen.

On the trail, allow nature to surround you. Let conversation fall away as the rhythm of walking quiets the mind. Silence frees you for internal communication and for connection with the world around you. Repeat an affirmation. Give thanks for strong legs, a healthy body, an opportunity to be outside.

Practice mindfulness by engaging all the senses. My mental routine on hikes carries me through a sensory cycle that increases my awareness of the surroundings. For a few minutes, I focus attention on what I see as I walk. Then I turn to another sense, paying attention to what I smell, what I feel, what I hear. Slowly, the series awakens me to nature. It pulls my attention to rustling leaves and the crack of a twig beneath my boot. It alerts me to the breeze that floats up from a creek. To the warm scent of sage in morning air.

Eventually, the rhythm of walking calms the mind and turns us inward. It restores connection with the soul and with harmonies best heard in silence. In those moments of union, we marvel at the velvet folds of a wild iris. We hear the question in a birdcall. A sense of connection with nature, of feeling that one is a part of a living cosmos, is a characteristic of spiritually healthy people, according to psychologist Marsha Sinetar,[9] author of *Ordinary People as Monks and Mystics*.

By quieting the mind and opening the senses, we invite opportunities to experience union with a vast network of life. One year when I found myself alone on Mother's Day, I took advantage of an unscheduled afternoon and stole away to a nearby county park. A gentle trail climbs one and a half miles from the parking lot to an open, rolling summit. The hike is easy but steady, ascending through grassy meadows and oak groves.

*I am here and I am breathing,* I reminded myself as I felt the familiar protests rise from my legs when my path turned up the hill. As I climbed, I encountered a pair of women descending the trail—a mother and daughter, I imagined, celebrating their kinship with a Mother's Day hike. The thought brought pleasure to my steps. Then it pulsed through my cells with a current of awareness that rippled my skin with goose bumps. In that instant I felt my kinship with the mother whose calm presence had drawn me here. The mother whose body supported my weight. Mother Earth. Provider of nourishment for body and soul. My throat tightened in an embrace of emotion: *I am here and I am walking with my Mother; I am here and I give thanks.*

Now each step connected me with an enormous sense of belonging. Each enveloped me in reassurance and safety. Then the moment passed like a gust of air that lifts the hair on my arms and drifts on. My steps continued to the grassy knoll where I strolled among other Sunday hikers and gazed at distant mountains. After a drink of water from my bottle, I turned and retraced my steps to the parking lot. By the time I reached the car, my mind had shifted into work mode, but beneath the thoughts of evening obligations and Monday commitments, a gentle warmth remained. It lingered in my cells like the tender caress of a caring mother.

## SACRED PLACES AND SPIRITUAL PATHS

Walking strengthens the physical balance of the body, bringing stability and coordination to our movement through life. Contact with nature balances the spirit, renewing emotional and spiritual resiliency. When we walk in nature, we experience an integration of the physical and spiritual frameworks that support our daily lives.

Psychological research suggests that simply spending thirty minutes alone each week in a natural setting provides significant therapeutic benefits for people.[10] Environmental psychologist James A. Swan says half an hour in nature gives us time to reconnect with our roots, with who and what we are. A thirty-minute hike done in silence and awareness points us forward in life with a renewed balance of internal and external energies.

A good hike encourages us to step back from the stresses and challenges of life for a few minutes or hours. It invites us to reconnect with the larger universe to which we belong. "Every landscape is a state of the soul, and who reads in both marvels at the likeness in every detail," a nineteenth-century Swiss walker wrote in his diary.[11] In the elegance of a mountain pine or boldness of a paintbrush blossom, we find reflections that wake us from mindless habits. We hear "aha's" that pull us back on course. Sometimes nature takes us by surprise, delivering a truth that resonates so loudly it echoes throughout our lives.

Adventurers recount "peak experiences," moments of ecstatic connection with the wonder and enormity of life. Spiritual travelers describe experiences of "ecstasy" and "rapture" when prayer or meditation delivers them into a sense of oneness with all creation. Athletes speak of being "in the zone" when mind and body click into joyous union.

Each is identifying an experience of wholeness that carries us beyond the "shoulds" and "can'ts" of daily patterns. Often these peak experiences stand out as significant turning points in people's lives, like the moment of joy that Margo Chisholm experienced at the top of Mount Kilimanjaro. They catch us off guard and vibrate through our cells. Often they occur in nature.

"What happens, I believe, is that nature affirms our identity. It shows us the spiritual dimensions of life, and that sets a baseline for the soul that can last a lifetime," Swan says. Peak experiences engulf us in a profound sense of connection with something greater than our mortal selves. All of us long for this kinship and for reassurance that we belong. When we find it, insecurity and fear vanish for a moment. We feel peace, joy, reverence, and awe. We experience bliss.

Moments of spiritual wholeness and connection aren't reserved for hikers, but many people find that such experiences occur more often and more easily in nature than elsewhere. Swan says that's because nature feeds a human hunger that religion may not satisfy. Religion nurtures spiritual community; nature fortifies the spirit. Nature keeps alive the intuitive senses that have sent mystics and seekers of all faiths into the wilderness to ask for guidance and vision. Today, the tradition survives in vision treks and nature retreats. It lives in the adventures of hikers and trekkers who travel the sacred contours of earth while exploring interior landscapes.

"The path is you," writes Buddhist monk Thich Nhat Hanh. "You will be like the tree of life. Your leaves, trunk, branches, and the blossoms of your soul will be fresh and beautiful, once you enter the practice of Earth Touching."[12]

Touching the earth as we walk keeps us in contact with the physical environment we live in. At the same time, we enter a magic kingdom that frees us from the constraints of daily life. Moving forward, one step at a time, we gradually

leave behind schedules, appointments, obligations. We surrender to the present moment, caught up in the beauty of
an inspiring vista or the demands of a rigorous climb. In
that surrender, we relax and open ourselves to the unexpected. We see the sacred in nature, and then sometimes in
ourselves.

On a spring hike into the red-rock majesty surrounding
Sedona, Arizona, my husband and I left the coolness of Oak
Creek Canyon one morning to climb the flanks of Wilson
Mountain. With each switchback, the trail brought us
closer to the clusters of red stone columns perched atop the
surrounding hills. Carved by centuries of weather and
water, the pillars stand like silent sentinels above the T-shirt
and trinket shops of the village below.

After two hours of steady climbing beneath a brilliant
sun, I peered at the rocks with squinted eyes and open
imagination. I envisioned clusters of red-rock observers,
huddled in silent supervision of this magnificent land. In
the mind-set of surrender that seems to evolve out of persistent uphill efforts, I began to view the columns as stat-
uesque people, molded from the same energy as me but in
a more enduring form. I wondered how the car-clogged
roads below looked to them. I wondered if they were
watching me.

My husband suggested a drink of water when I pointed
out the watchers to him. Perhaps I'd had too much sun, he
joked. Perhaps the heat and the hype surrounding Sedona's
power spots had hurled me into a visual vortex. We laughed
and paused in the shade of a small tree to pull out the water
bottle.

Just beyond the tree, previous travelers had constructed a rock cairn, a pile of stones to mark the route to the summit. When we stepped forward into the final segment of our climb, a sense of well-being accompanied me. It warmed me like the April sun that wrapped around my shoulders. It blessed me with a red-rock benediction, a sense of family all around me in the wilderness.

# From Sole to Soul . . .

*Sacred Paces:* Travel to distant mountains if you wish. Seek out the sacred grounds of ancient peoples if you can. But when lack of time or money keeps you closer to home, let yourself explore the sacred places right around the corner in parks and parking lots. No matter where you walk or live, sacred space is as close as your front door.

"Whoever you are: some evening take a step out of your house, which you know so well. Enormous space is near," wrote the poet Rainer Maria Rilke.[13] We can find that space by opening our senses and setting forth with an attitude of expectancy. Expect the sacred and we enter it.

Step onto the path of a spiritual traveler by walking city streets or neighborhood parks with the reverence you would take to a shrine. Make a gesture of respect by picking up one piece of litter—one candy wrapper, one cigarette butt, one soda can. Make a gift of awareness by opening your senses and reconnecting with a route you've grown numb to. Give thanks for the steady strength of a single tree rising from a city courtyard. Acknowledge the vivid blue of the sky, the red of an awning, the music floating from an open window.

So often we walk in mindless detachment from the world around us. We hurry from parking lots to offices without noticing a single thing along the way. We save our sense of wonder and awe for special occasions or famous destinations. We long for reminders of life's miracles and lose touch with the wonder we pass everyday. We forget that the route to sacred places always leads through the mind and soul. Recognition depends on awareness and vision. The sacred simply waits for us to notice.

*Rules of Thumb:* In traditional forms of sitting meditation, people often position their hands in a particular way. Some meditators make a circle of the thumb and middle finger of each hand. Some cup their hands in the lap with thumbs touching. These hand positions are called *mudras* in Sanskrit and are often used in Buddhist art as an outward representation of an inner state of being.

An adaptation of these mudras can be useful on hikes when heat, fatigue, or a difficult trail challenge both your inner and outer being. If a long hike stretches into a warm afternoon, it's common to experience swelling in the hands. This exercise helps reduce the swelling by exercising the fingers. It also gives the mind a physical backup for affirmations that keep you moving.

Bend the arms and hold your hands at about waist height. Cup the fingers gently and form a circle with the thumb and forefinger of each hand. Beginning with thumb and forefinger, tap the thumb lightly against the tip of each finger as if running a scale to the little finger and back again. Synchronize each tap with a step.

Now add a melody. With each tap, recite this refrain: One-step-for-ward-at-a-time. (Pause.) One-step-for-ward-at-a-time. The words are magical. They remind you to stay in the moment instead of fretting about how long the hike has been and how far you still have to go.

Change the words and the mudra if you wish. Tap twice on each finger or alter the sequence. Just keep it simple and steady to accompany your steps. The phrase suggested here creates an eight-step pattern with the pause. If you use this pattern for long periods of time, skip a beat occasionally so that you change the foot you begin on. Generally, people land more heavily on the exhale than on the inhale. Simply by rotating the lead foot from time to time, you balance the physical and psychological impact of stepping forward. The subtle integration of breath and movement provides a practice of flexibility that increases stability and ease on either foot.

# CHAPTER 10

## On the Pilgrim's Path
### STEPPING OUT WITH PURPOSE

We'd been walking for three days by the time we reached the New Dungeon Ghyll Hotel. Our steps had traversed hillsides seamed with stacked-stone walls and had roused the hollow gaze of black-faced Herdwick sheep. Each day had moved us deeper into the green core of the English Lake District. Each distanced us from the tea shops and inns of lakeside villages that hummed with the commerce of tour-bus travelers.

Our route skirted the country home of Beatrix Potter, where lines of tourists wrapped around the garden fence. It bypassed the cottage of poet William Wordsworth. Our destination lay in the craggy wilderness of the Langdale Pikes. We advanced toward it in silence now. Three days of walking had exhausted our need for commentary on the landscape, the sheep, or the weather. Trail signs no longer sent us into debate. By now, we had learned that "pike" and "fell" mean mountain in this northern corner of England where Old Norse still rules place names. "Ghyll" identifies a tumbling mountain stream; "tarn" means mountain lake.

These first days had been a warm-up for the steeper slopes awaiting us on a ten-day trek through England's most popular national park. Novelist Daniel Defoe once dismissed these hills as high and formidable, with "a kind of unhospitable terror in them . . . all barren and wild, of no use or advantage either to man or beast."[1]

Almost three hundred years later, the advantage has grown more obvious. Eighteen hundred miles of hiking trails lace the region, welcoming refugees from lives tamed by progress.[2] Here, walkers retreat into the forces of nature on day hikes or long-distance treks. Three companions and I planned to cover 130 miles of the network on a self-guided walk from inn to inn. We booked rooms in advance and departed from Windermere with only the clothing, maps, and guidebooks we could stuff into large daypacks.

When we arrived at the New Dungeon Ghyll Hotel, we spread detailed quarter-section maps on a table outside the pub. We peered up from our lager at trails gouged into the flanks of the mountains before us. The next morning we breakfasted on Cumberland sausage and broiled tomatoes before shrugging our packs into place and pushing our bodies up the slope behind the hotel.

Lake District routes tend to shun the frivolity of switchbacks or traverses, and our trail made no exception. The way led straight up the fall line in a relentless slog that quickly silenced morning banter. For more than an hour, we scrambled along the rocky edge of Dungeon Ghyll, a thin cascade of tumbling water. We found its source at the top of the climb. The waters of Stickle Tarn shimmered in a rocky basin below a sheer rock face. We paused to unfold the map once more and reconfirm our route.

While we rested, clouds slid over the ragged crest that towered above the lake. A thick fog unfolded over us. We pulled on Gore-Tex and fortified ourselves with chocolate-covered graham crackers. Then we turned away from the lake and followed the track across a boggy highland heath. Mists floated beside us, cloaking us in isolation one moment and lifting the next to reveal craggy mysteries. Rocky buttresses protruded from the moors, desolate and beautiful at the same time. I walked with awe and with a hint of wariness. This landscape could have been the surface of the moon. Or a movie set. It seemed like a different world.

Later, I understood that it was. On this cryptic ridge, I had stepped across a boundary. I'd reached the timeless present—a place that often seems as distant from my life as the planet Mars. Here, the uphill scramble was forgotten. The days ahead fell from view. Nothing intruded on the magic of this moment. Nothing detracted from an enchanting landscape where streamers of cloud dipped and rose in a silken flow. In moments of opening, I took bearings on the formations ahead. When filmy isolation swallowed me again, I'd peer into the softness for cues, delighting in the cycle of obscurity and vision. I had reached the place of joyous freedom that I'd come looking for.

More than adventure, challenge, or connection with nature, this is the target my steps seek, no matter what landscape I travel. Long walks lift the constraints of schedules. They loosen the shackles of compulsion and control. They carry travelers into a world with no flights to catch, no meters to feed. Nothing to do but connect with the present, one step at a time.

This freedom isn't hard to find once you start walking, but getting there usually takes a few days. After three and a half days, my body and mind have slowed to a pace that gives me time to forget about time. On an English moor, I have fallen into stride with writer Peter Matthiessen, trekking the highlands of Nepal twenty-two years and a continent away: "gradually, my mind has cleared itself, and wind and sun pour through my head, as through a bell. Though we talk little here, I am never lonely; I am returned into myself," he wrote in *The Snow Leopard,* an account of his 1973 journey in the Himalayas.[3]

Peace of mind is a quiet destination. Lost in the rhythms of steady walking, I rarely notice when I've arrived. Instead, I enter the world of paradox that long walks frequently explore. By distancing myself from familiar settings and patterns, I have closed a gap inside myself. A few days of walking have brought me back home, returned to a condition of completeness where nothing more is needed. Right now, I am enough; I have enough.

"To glimpse one's own true nature is a kind of home-going, . . . the homegoing that needs no home," Matthiessen concurs.[4] Sometimes a homesickness for this place of silent contentment sweeps through me at unexpected moments: in a bustling café where too many people are talking at once; at a symphony, when I feel a sudden impulse to curl up in the peace behind the notes. Memories linger in my cells like snapshots in a family album.

All travel lifts us out of numbing patterns and introduces new points of view. It brings shifts in attitude and aware-ness. But not all travel is equal. Travelers who venture forth on foot find that walking makes a world of difference. On foot, the journey becomes the destination. "Where" matters less than "why."

## AFOOT ON THE CAUSEWAY

"A pilgrim is a wanderer with a purpose," wrote a woman who walked twenty-five thousand miles and never lost sight of why. "My walking is first of all a prayer for peace," she told reporters, civic groups, and curious observers who marveled at a silver-haired matron traveling on foot alone.[5] Peace Pilgrim believed that inner peace was the first step in achieving world peace. Walking was her path to inner peace. Where she traveled mattered little. Why she walked was never in doubt.

"A pilgrimage can be to a place—that's the best known kind—but it can also be for a thing. Mine is for peace," she said.[6] "When I started out on my pilgrimage, I was using walking for two purposes. . . . One was to contact people . . . but the other was as a prayer discipline. To keep me concentrated on my prayer for peace. My personal prayer is: Make me an instrument through which only truth can speak."[7] At the time of her death in 1981, Peace Pilgrim was completing her seventh trek across the United States.

Many modern pilgrims have traveled the same route, crossing states and mountain ranges to make coast-to-coast declarations of beliefs. In recent decades, cross-country walkers have called attention to political, medical, and environmental issues. Their steps demonstrate a commitment to making a difference in the world.

Instead of walking across the country, surgeon Gordon Klatt decided to circle the clock in support of his convictions. On a college track near his home in Tacoma, Washington, he undertook a twenty-four-hour endurance test to raise awareness and funds for cancer research. Several years of medical practice had led him into the personal lives of cancer patients and their families as a compassionate physician. Now he wanted to do more.

For eighteen hours he alternated a lap of walking with a lap of jogging around the track. Then his legs began to disappear. It felt as if he were moving on sticks. Movement slowed to a steady walk. For six more hours he held the course. "I used visionary techniques," he says.[8] "I imagined what it would be like at the end, to finish after twenty-four hours."

On the sidelines, friends and community members cheered him on. They counted the laps as he went by. Many had pledged financial contributions for each mile he com-

# Side Lines

## SPIRITUAL JOURNEYS FOR WALKERS AND PILGRIMS

Eight hundred years ago, half a million travelers a year followed the Way of Saint James to Santiago de Compostela in Spain.[9] At the height of the popularity of religious pilgrimage, two hundred thousand pilgrims a year traveled to the shrine of Saint Thomas à Becket in Canterbury, England.[10]

Those traditional routes draw a different pilgrim today. Recreational travelers who seek both adventure and renewal follow historic trails around the globe to connect with past and present. Guidebooks and tour companies offer extensive information about many long-distance excursions, including these well-traveled paths:

*Camino de Santiago (The Way of Saint James), Spain:* The first travel guide to this pilgrimage across northern Spain from the French border to the city of Santiago de Compostela was written in about 1150 A.D.[11] Charlemagne and Saint Francis of Assisi are said to have been among the millions of pilgrims drawn to the tomb of Saint James.[12] Disputes about the authenticity of the saint's remains have not dulled pilgrims' dedication to the route throughout the centuries.

Contemporary walkers complete the five-hundred-mile trek in about a month, averaging twenty miles a day and staying in small inns or spreading sleeping bags on bunks in rustic *refugios*. A shortened version on the ninety-mile final stretch from Cebreiro can be accomplished in five days.

*The Canterbury Trail, Canterbury, England:* When Thomas à Becket, archbishop of Canterbury, was murdered inside Canterbury Cathedral by followers of Henry II, Canterbury became the most holy shrine in Great Britain. Becket's death in 1170 roused such a furor that even Henry II donned sackcloth in 1174 to make the 130-mile pilgrimage as a penance.

Today, much of the route follows the North Downs Way, a long-distance footpath that travels through farmlands and villages. Although Chaucer's pilgrims set out from London in the fourteenth-century *Canterbury Tales,* the traditional starting point was Winchester, a center of travel and trade in southern England.[13]

*The Royal Incan Road, Machu Picchu, Peru:* A five-day trek along an ancient roadway in the Peruvian Andes has become a popular pilgrimage for modern walkers. The journey from Cuzco to the spectacular Incan citadel of Machu Picchu carries hikers into the hub of the Incan empire along segments of a road that once extended 3,250 miles from Ecuador to Argentina.[14]

The fifty-mile segment from Cuzco rises to an elevation of 13,780 feet and then descends to the ruins of Machu Picchu at 8,200 feet. Archaeologists date construction of the Incan Road and Machu Picchu in the 1400s.

*The Appalachian National Scenic Trail, Eastern United States:* The 2,144-mile Appalachian National Scenic Trail was the first federally protected footpath in the United States. The route travels through fourteen states, stretching from Springer Mountain in Georgia to Mount Katahdin in Maine, along a path constructed between 1921 and 1937.[15]

Hikers who tackle the full trail typically commit five or six months to the journey, traveling the eastern ridges of the United States with tents and sleeping bags. The route carries them through a scenic corridor that includes two national parks, eight national forests, and two national historic parks.

Hundreds of access trails along the route allow walkers with less time to enjoy hikes of almost any distance and difficulty. On some sections of the trail, proximity to villages makes inn-to-inn hiking an attractive option.

pleted. Some pledged more than money. They backed his vision with medical assistance, food, encouragement, and occasional companionship on the track during a grueling journey that brought him to the starting line 328 times.

When the countdown stopped at twenty-four hours, he'd traveled a total of eighty-two miles around the oval, a distance greater than three marathons done back-to-back. The journey led him to an unplanned destination—it took him into the national spotlight. On the strength of a vision and a commitment, Gordon Klatt had raised $27,000 for the American Cancer Society and demonstrated the difference one person can make by stepping forward. Almost two million people in communities across the country now circle local tracks in Relay for Life events inspired by his example. The twenty-four-hour effort that Gordon launched in 1985 has ballooned into the major fund-raising activity of the American Cancer Society. And it hasn't lost a healing focus.

Those who come in memory of loved ones share the track with those who walk in celebration of survival. Professionals shed roles that isolate them. Most walk on relay teams, alternating the laps with colleagues, neighbors, friends. Together, they circle toward the catharsis that arises from long walks and deep commitment. "There is a good feeling that comes from that," Gordon says. "I think it is a very therapeutic event."

Some would say that Gordon's twenty-four-hour journey on a college track contains the classic components of pilgrimage: surrender, sacrifice, and service. Preparation exacted a year of training, organizing, and arm-twisting. Recovery claimed another three months. Benefits extended to millions of people and have spanned a dozen years.

In traditional interpretations, a pilgrimage is a journey on a sacred path, to a sacred place, for a sacred goal. For thousands of years, religious pilgrims have traveled to the shrines of saints and deities around the globe. Almost every major religion has given rise to some form of pilgrimage. Birthplaces, burial sites, hallowed groves, and sacred grottoes surround a pantheon of spiritual practices. Believers undergo the hardships of pilgrimage as an act of devotion or perhaps penance. The journey manifests an appeal to higher powers for healing, pardon, or spiritual merit.

And perhaps the parallel goes further. Gordon's demanding trek around the clock wound up exactly where it started. Both the track and the timepiece mark start and finish at the same place. Each revolution brings one back to the beginning. Moving forward requires starting over. Paradox, religious scholars say, is another classic component of pilgrimage. When the body grows heavy with fatigue, the soul becomes light. When feet find connection with the earth, the spirit begins to fly. Traveling to a distant shrine leads a traveler home.

## ONE PILGRIM'S PROGRESS

When James Carse set out to walk five hundred miles from the French border to the coast of Spain, his footsteps formed a deep and immediate connection with the earth. Day after day he slogged through mud and dung on the historic Camino de Santiago. Relentless rains converted the Way of Saint James into the way of surrender long before it approached the cathedral at Santiago de Compostela, which has attracted pilgrims since the Middle Ages.

Water breached the resistant surface of his rain gear and filled the pores of an inner fleece jacket. It spilled along his skin. Ankle-deep muck overflowed the tops of his trail boots. Each step mired him down. One day brought an outbreak of snails so pervasive he couldn't move without the awful crunch of shells. Disagreeable, yes, but he never thought of giving up. Instead, he simply gave in.

"Sometimes it got so funny I'd laugh out loud at the water pouring down and inside me. I was totally soaked, and there was a kind of security in it. In some ways, I really got to enjoy it. It's like you sometimes feel around a fire in the evening when a snowstorm is raging," he recalls.[16]

At the end of a twenty-mile day, he'd seek the comfort of small inns along the ancient pilgrimage route. He'd sit by a fire to dry his pants and wipe mud from his shoes. It often took an hour to clean and bandage blistered feet after walking all day with wet socks. He'd glance up from the task at travelers who arrived at the door in cars. They'd dash through the entry shaking umbrellas and grimacing in disgust. Watching them, he felt an odd comfort.

"I didn't really need those cars or that kind of protection. Somehow, you had the feeling you didn't have to run for shelter. You somehow find a shelter from within. It was just part of the path. You have to accept that."

Writer and professor emeritus of religion at New York University, Carse undertook the twenty-seven-day trek from the Pyrenees to the Atlantic not to honor the apostle James, whose bones legend places in the Cathedral of Santiago de Compostela. He walked in memory of a woman he met in divinity school and who shared his path for thirty-seven years. As she approached death, his wife asked him to use her savings to stretch himself, to do something that expanded his spiritual life. A practiced hiker, walker, and meditator, he chose a solitary trek on an historic route. He undertook a private pilgrimage.

"I knew about the pilgrimage historically and thought I would do it as a reflective experience," he says. He equipped for the outing with a daypack for underwear, socks, and maps. He arrived with an attitude of willingness, trusting the trek to lead him somewhere, but he didn't know where that would be. "I knew this was just the sort of experience Alice had in mind for me: a physically and spiritually challenging journey into the unfamiliar. From these efforts you get things you couldn't have imagined anyway."

The Camino de Santiago did not disappoint him. In spite of rains that dampened two out of every three days, Carse felt his spirits lifting. The road led him over mountain ridges where rain turned to snow and into hostels so cold he slept between mattresses. Almost daily, he missed a marker and extended his route by getting lost. It was grim sometimes, but it was also triumphant.

When skies cleared, he looked ahead to the spires of village churches marking his path in the distance. He followed them through fields of sunflowers and into vineyards fragrant with October harvests. Striding full-out down a stretch of country road, he'd cruise into a blissful zone where he felt he could go on forever. Felt exuberant and alive.

"I had gone to think things over, and instead, I didn't think at all," he says. "Your attention is absorbed most effectively by things of an immediate nature—you think about your feet, or you study the map for the fifty-third time in an afternoon. Then you've gone miles and you can't remember a thing that happened. It was cleansing in a surprising way. It was like *no* experience. You just do it. You don't much think about it. In a certain way, it was rather ecstatic."

The blissful mindlessness that settles into the body of a long-distance walker rises from attitude, not scenery or destination. It matters not whether trails lead to shrines or to waterfalls when the walker sets out with willingness to see the journey through. Bliss even turns up on fragmented jaunts that stop in the middle of nowhere. Walking across the United States one week at a time on an installment plan that stretched over a decade, singer Art Garfunkel exalted in the same tranquillity. "By the third day, mile number thirty-five, lost in isolation, the body feels Zen-pleasurable," he told a reporter after completing a segment in Montana.[17]

## A Pocketful of Prayer Stones

When travel provides a metaphor, any trek that connects a walker with what is sacred can be called a pilgrimage. Every nature walk, every weekend hike, even lunch-hour strolls in the park provide a kind of pilgrimage when walkers infuse their excursions with the reverence that pilgrims bring to sacred paths. Those who seek connection with something greater than themselves can find it, no matter what the route.

In mountain passes of Nepal, travelers attach prayer flags to bamboo poles and hoist them into the wind. On gusty summits, the flags flap into the sky tossing petitions and praises to the gods who reside in surrounding mountains. In the New Mexico village of Chimayó, supplicants rub the powdery soil of the Sangre de Cristo foothills on imperfect bodies and seek the miracle of healing from the sacred land. In Great Britain, visitors at ancient Celtic sites dip holy water from sacred wells in tribute to the life-giving liquid that flows from the ground.

"Behind nature, throughout nature, spirit is present," confirms essayist Ralph Waldo Emerson.[18] "Nature is made to conspire with spirit to emancipate us."[19] Walking encourages intimacy with nature and with ourselves, connecting us with that which is divine in both. Any long-distance walk will probably get you there, but those who enter nature seeking wholeness and holiness approach as pilgrims.

In the Lake District of northern England, I finger the agate pebbles in my pocket and thank the energies of nature that heal the splits in me. The agates come from the coast of

Oregon, picked up in walks along the edge of breakers. These stones connect me with my origins. They hold a family history of seeking comfort in the ocean's ebb and flow. On treks, I carry them with me the way other pilgrims might carry prayer beads, *milagros,* saints' medals, or incense.

The custom has followed me from the highlands of Nepal. In a roadless region bordered by mountains, treasures from the sea evoke awe. Shells that wash against the shores of my home without notice come to rest on altars there. They connect the mountains and the sea. They affirm a world that can't be seen.

These pebbles do the same for me. They connect me with a world that can only be found with an open heart. When I hike, I leave one on a mountain ridge or in the dry bed of a desert stream. The practice has grown into a ritual, a gesture of gratitude to the spirit that connects earth and sea and me. The gift is insignificant; the intention transforms every hike into a pilgrimage.

The ritual of giving heightens awareness of what is sought. It acknowledges what has been received. A gift compounds the parallels between long walks and pilgrimage. In some cultures, offerings of cornmeal, salt, flowers, or incense acknowledge the omnipresent power of nature. Modern pilgrims can make a gift of service, picking up litter that is found on a trail or showing respect for the environment by sticking a baggie in your pocket to carry out your own orange peels and toilet paper, a generous act that honors both nature and fellow walkers.

Such gestures of respect distinguish pilgrims from tourists, says James Swan, author of *Sacred Places.* A tourist goes to nature for recreation, seeking views and experiences that are pleasing to the senses. A pilgrim looks to nature for re-creation, a deeper experience that nourishes both the senses and the soul.[20] Mindfulness characterizes a pilgrim, regardless of the path or destination. It's not where you go but how you get there that makes life a pilgrimage.

Before we dip below the English mists and descend into the next valley, I pull a stone from my pocket and drop it into the cradle of a rock crevice. It slips from my fingers with a silent "thank you" and tumbles through a riff of lauds: *I give thanks for the wonder of this place. I give thanks for strong legs, good health, and curiosity. I give thanks for the joy in my life.*

Gently I lift a fist to my chest and tap it over my heart. The gesture sends a thank-you to the spirit within, acknowledging the part of me that in this glorious moment finds the sacred in everything. It vibrates in my soul. To see the sacred in all its forms, both common and mysterious—this is the soul's gift of vision. No words are needed here, just a pebble and a touch. Enchantment envelops me. My spirit soars in gratitude for journeys that slow me down, for walks that lead me where I want to go on the pilgrimage that is my life.

Slowly the vibrations subside and silence washes through me again. Sensation dissolves into the vastness of oneness. I am at home. I am at peace.

# From Sole to Soul . . .

*A Grateful Retreat:* Spiritual retreats provide a temporary withdrawal from everyday life. They create islands of peace and contemplation that restore body and spirit, preparing us to return to the world refreshed and energized. Typically, retreat is a time of silence, of stilling external noises in order to hear the higher wisdom of an inner voice. This exercise invites you to step away from your usual patterns and obligations for a mini-retreat of two or three hours. Commit to do it without conversation or unnecessary talking.

Prepare yourself for the retreat by selecting a location. Perhaps you already have a favorite walking path along the river or through an arboretum. Choose a park or nature area convenient to your home. Even a neighborhood pocket park will suffice. Cemeteries can be peaceful and quiet. Then prepare the items you'll take on your retreat. Decide on a small gift or offering to leave in appreciation—a stone or shell or a few grains of salt. Put your gift in a daypack with a bottle of water, a notebook and pen, and something to sit on if you need it. If you wish, take along something that symbolizes spirit to you. It could be an object, a picture, a poem.

If you are driving to your retreat location, begin the silence in the car. No radio. No singing. No shouting at other drivers. If you can walk to the park or trail, begin the retreat when you leave home.

223

Part One—Thirty Minutes: Walk in silence for thirty minutes. Walk at a moderate pace and begin to still the mind by focusing on your breathing. Count your steps as you inhale and exhale. Think about the air moving in and out of your body, drawing in renewal and releasing stagnation. Keep your eyes on the ground ahead of you and let your focus soften slightly. In traditional walking meditations, students often walk back and forth on a path or go around a garden loop. You don't need to get anyplace with this walk. Simply walk and continue to bring the focus back to your breathing and your footsteps.

Part Two—Fifteen Minutes: Find a place where you will feel comfortable sitting for fifteen minutes. Settle in and take a couple of deep breaths. Keeping your eyes lowered, turn your attention to listening. What sounds do you hear nearby? Traffic noises? Rustling leaves? Birds? Children at a playground? Focus on each sound for a minute, intentionally isolating what you hear. Slowly move your range of hearing farther out. Can you hear music from a distant radio? The voices of other walkers? Listening meditations prepare us to observe and hear with intention and increased clarity. Usually we are so occupied with the chatter in our heads that we are unable to give full attention to anything else. Intentional listening provides practice in shutting off internal babble and helps sharpen awareness.

Part Three—Thirty Minutes: Walk in awareness and gratitude. As you resume your meditative walking pace, become aware of all your senses and of the information that surrounds you. Notice what you see, hear, feel, smell. Identify the sensations mentally. *I see sunlight reflecting on the river. I hear someone talking.* Gradually let your awareness guide you to something you are grateful for. *I hear a bird chirping: I am thankful for the sounds of nature. I hear a car horn: I am thankful for this sanctuary in the midst of traffic.* Let the exercise become a free association of awareness and gratitude so that your appreciation flows from what you are noticing: *I feel a cold wind: I am grateful for a warm jacket; I am grateful for changing seasons. I see a candy wrapper on the ground: I am thankful for a flexible back that lets me bend over to pick it up; I am grateful to the crews who maintain this area. I see shadows on the sidewalk: I am grateful for light and dark; I am grateful for the coolness of shade.* When some part of your mind gets bored and wanders off, bring it back to the present and to your senses as you continue the walking meditation.

Part Four—Fifteen Minutes: Write it down. Return to your sitting spot, or select another location where you can write for fifteen minutes. What did you notice about your awareness and gratitude in the past thirty minutes? Did you surprise yourself? Are there things you found it difficult to regard with gratitude? Did you find one sense easier to notice than others? When you complete your notes, say thank you to your surroundings for the awareness you gained by walking here. Perhaps one thought stands out for you. Acknowledge that with appreciation. Leave your gift here, or if another spot seems significant, walk to that location and express your appreciation during the next walking segment.

Part Five—Thirty Minutes: Walk in silence. To clear the mind and release thoughts that have followed you from the writing, return to the breath awareness that you practiced in the first period of walking. Simply focus on the breath moving in and out of your body. Count your footsteps and let go of all thoughts. Gradually move your awareness to your footsteps. Feel your heel touch the ground and imagine that your foot is sinking into the earth, planting peace with each step. Leave an impression of gratitude in the soil. If you have not left your gift yet, do that before you leave the retreat area. Acknowledge yourself for devoting two hours to a spiritual practice that has carried you deeper into yourself.

If you can commit more than two hours to the retreat, lengthen the segments, or repeat each of them. If you have less time, shorten the walking periods to twenty minutes. Even a lunch-hour break allows time to retreat with Parts One and Two. Because we have grown accustomed to hearing music in elevators and grocery stores and to the sound of televisions blaring around the clock, silence can feel awkward at first.

Trappist monk Thomas Merton, a prolific writer and advocate of solitude, acknowledged that not everyone is called to be a hermit or a monk. Nevertheless, all people "need enough silence and solitude in their lives to enable the deep inner voice of their own true self to be heard at least occasionally," he advised.[21]

Be patient and you will find that silence is restorative to body and mind. Even an hour or two of silence allows us to feel more centered and clear. It opens a channel to the soul.

# BOOKS AND RESOURCES

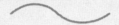

A number of fitness-walking books cover the basic physical considerations of setting up a successful walking exercise program and supplement the spiritual-mental focus of *The Spirited Walker*. Some feature specialized techniques such as racewalking. Others explore the pleasures of trail walking. As you read additional materials about walking, you constantly build awareness and skill. You also deepen your commitment to a healthy walking practice.

## WALKING TECHNIQUES AND WORKOUTS

**Bricklin, Mark, and Maggie Spilner.** *Prevention's Practical Encyclopedia of Walking for Health.* Emmaus, PA: Rodale Press, 1992. This outstanding all-around walking guide covers walking from A to Z. Its accessible style and extensive coverage stretches from technique to footwear and even includes suggestions for walking meditation as a stress-reduction tool.

**Fenton, Mark, and Seth Bauer.** *The Ninety-Day Fitness Walking Program.* New York: Berkley, 1995. Written by the editors of *Walking* magazine, this book takes a get-started approach for people who have not been regular exercisers. It emphasizes the physical benefits of walking and is arranged in a day-by-day program that guides beginners from ten-minute strolls to thirty-minute walks.

**Ikonian, Therese.** *Fitness Walking.* Champaign, IL: Human Kinetics, 1995. Ikonian is a racewalker and walking instructor whose book moves quickly from walking basics to programs for advanced walkers. The core of the book is devoted to sample workouts for walkers at six fitness levels, allowing walkers to create training schedules that offer variety and increasing challenge.

**Smith, Kathy, with Susanna Levin.** *WALKFIT for a Better Body.* New York: Warner Books, 1994. All the basics are spelled out here for someone getting started on a walking program. Smith includes sections on stretching and weight workouts that complement an aerobic walking program.

**Snowdon, Les, and Maggie Humphreys.** *Walk Aerobics.* Woodstock, NY: Overlook Press, 1996. This fine guide to fitness walking, by the authors of *The Walking Diet*, addresses physical aspects of walking from calluses to calories. It recommends "inner walking" for relaxation and spiritual fitness.

## FITNESS, FLEXIBILITY, AND WELL-BEING

**Al Huang, Chungliang, and Jerry Lynch.** *Thinking Body, Dancing Mind: TaoSports for Extraordinary Performance in Athletics, Business, and Life*. New York: Bantam Books, 1992. Paperback edition, 1994. TaoSport incorporates Eastern spiritual philosophy with Western athletic performance. This book makes a strong connection between mental focus and peak athletic performance, identifying all physical action as a mind-body effort.

**Alter, Michael J.** *Sport Stretch*. Champaign, IL: Leisure Press, 1990. Alter provides very reliable information with solid anatomical explanations. Stretching is only good when you stretch properly, he advises. Illustrations and instructions accompany his suggestions.

**Anderson, Bob.** *Stretching*. Bolinas, CA: Shelter Publications, 1980. A thorough guide to stretching as a component of fitness. Anderson gives clear instructions on how and when to stretch and provides set groups of stretches to complement a variety of sports activities including walking.

**Benson, Herbert, and Marg Stark.** *Timeless Healing: The Power and Biology of Belief.* New York: Scribner, 1996. This work from the author of *The Relaxation Response* adds the element of faith to the formula of simple meditation that

Benson proposes as an antidote for many stress-related illnesses. Benson's studies show that jogging and walking can be as effective as sitting meditation is in triggering the benefits of mental relaxation.

**Murphy, Shane.** *The Achievement Zone: Eight Skills for Winning All the Time from the Playing Field to the Boardroom.* New York: Putnam, 1996. As sport psychologist to the U.S. Olympic Committee for seven years, Murphy worked with America's elite athletes and discovered that mental training was just as important as physical preparation. This book offers insights into mental and emotional skills that underlie success in any endeavor—physical, professional, or personal.

## IN THE COMPANY OF WALKERS

**Fletcher, Colin.** *The Secret Worlds of Colin Fletcher.* New York: Knopf, 1989. Author of *The Complete Walker,* an essential reference for backpackers, the venerable Colin Fletcher is a knowledgeable hiker and an entertaining writer. In *Secret Worlds,* he reflects on some of his favorite walks in chapters that reveal with humor and awe the rewards and challenges that draw walkers into nature. Entertaining and inspiring.

**Strickland, Ron,** ed. *Shank's Mare.* New York: Paragon House, 1988. From garden strolls to rugged expeditions, this collection of walking stories from travel journals, literature, and essays makes great bedtime reading for walkers. The anthology features works by twentieth-century writers, explorers, politicians, and adventurers who take time to observe life on foot.

Many walkers have recorded distance walks that make inspiring reading. Author Peter Matthiessen's trekking classic, *The Snow Leopard* (New York: Bantam Books, 1979), tracks his spiritual journey in the Himalayas and exposes the heart of Tibetan Buddhism within an elegant exploration of self. Peter Jenkins walks across the United States and encounters a vast internal and external geography in *A Walk Across America* (New York: Fawcett, 1983). Travel writer Bruce Chatwin spins extraordinarily entertaining tales of long walks and mindfulness. Try *In Patagonia* (New York: Summit Books, 1977) or *The Songlines* (New York: Viking, 1987).

## ON A SPIRITUAL PATH

**Easwaran, Eknath.** *Meditation: An Eight-Point Program.* Petaluma, CA: Nilgiri Press, 1978. Written by the founder of Blue Mountain Center of Meditation and a former Fulbright professor at the University of California at Berkeley, this book introduces a method of meditation that uses inspirational passages to focus the mind. It is gentle and down-to-earth in outlining a way of life that enriches daily experiences.

**Hanh, Thich Nhat.** *The Long Road Turns to Joy: A Guide to Walking Meditation.* Berkeley, CA: Parallax Press, 1996. A Buddhist monk, poet, and peace activist, the author invites walkers to make each step a meditation. This pocket-sized book introduces traditional Zen walking meditation with eloquent simplicity and clarity.

**Housden, Roger.** *Retreats.* San Francisco: HarperSanFrancisco, 1995. From a walk in the woods to a month of Zen meditation, the spiritual value of a retreat from daily life becomes clear in this beautiful guide. With photographs and descriptions, the book provides a broad introduction to religions, institutions, retreat centers, and travel services that encourage spiritual retreats.

**Mundy, Linus.** *Prayer-Walking.* St. Meinrad, IN: Abbey Press, 1994. Reissued as *The Complete Guide to Prayer Walking* (New York: Crossroad, 1996). This inviting pocket guide encourages "taking a stroll with your soul" by reciting Christian prayers and scriptures while walking.

## RESOURCES

The American Volksport Association sponsors noncompetitive ten-kilometer walks around the country. These low-key events welcome individuals and families of all ages and walking speeds. Local chapters often include fitness-walking groups that meet regularly between events. For information about clubs in your area, contact American Volksport Association, 1001 Pat Booker Road, Suite 101, Universal City, TX 78148 (1–800–830–9255).

The YMCA Walk Reebok program offers encouragement and instruction for walkers with a variety of fitness goals. Trained instructors coordinate workouts for three groups of walkers: health walkers, who maintain a leisurely walking pace; fitness walkers who move at a pace of thirteen to fifteen minutes per mile; and speed walkers, who push to hit a twelve-minute-mile pace. Call your local YMCA to see if the program is available in your community or to request that it be added to offerings.

For information about racewalking clubs and coaches throughout the United States, contact the North American Racewalking Foundation, P. O. Box 50312, Pasadena, CA 91115–0312 (1–818–577–2264).

Sports Music Incorporated produces workout music on tape and CD. The collections are programmed to satisfy a wide range of musical tastes and walking speeds. Many tapes include vocal music, but a few all-instrumental programs are suitable background for spirited walkers. For a catalog, call 1–800–878–4764 or write Sports Music, Box 769689, Roswell, GA 30076.

*Walking* magazine provides a steady source of information and inspiration in six issues a year. Pick up a copy at a newsstand or call for subscription information: 1–800–829–5585 in the U.S. and Canada.

*Prevention* magazine presents walking news and tips in the "Walker's World" section of each issue and in an informative quarterly newsletter for members of the Prevention Walking Club. Check issues of the monthly magazine for information on the club, or contact Prevention Walking Club: 1–800–666–1216.

# NOTES

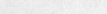

## INTRODUCTION

1. Dorothy Gilman, *A New Kind of Country* (Garden City, NY: Doubleday, 1978), 123.
2. Michael Murphy and Rhea A. White, *In the Zone* (New York: Penguin Books, 1995), 1–6. Originally published as *The Psychic Side of Sports* (Reading, MA: Addison-Wesley, 1978).

## CHAPTER 1

1. Henry David Thoreau, "Walking," *Atlantic Monthly*, vol. 9, no. 56 (June 1862): 659.
2. Thoreau, "Walking," *Atlantic Monthly*, vol. 9, no. 56 (June 1862): 657.
3. Benefits of walking and meditation derived from Herbert Benson, with Marg Stark, *Timeless Healing: The Power and Biology of Belief*

(New York: Scribner, 1996); Benson, with Miriam Z. Klipper, *The Relaxation Response* (New York: Morrow, 1975); Mark Bricklin and Maggie Spilner, *Prevention's Practical Encyclopedia of Walking for Health* (Emmaus, PA: Rodale Press, 1992); James M. Rippe, "Let's Get Moving—Start Walking!," *Newsweek,* vol. 125., no. 9, Feb. 27, 1995, special advertising section; "Physical Activity and Public Health: A Recommendation from the Centers for Disease Control and Prevention and the American College of Sports Medicine," *Journal of the American Medical Association* 273, no. 5 (Feb. 1, 1995): 402; Gary Yanker and Kathy Burton (with a team of fifty medical experts), *Walking Medicine: The Lifetime Guide to Preventive and Rehabilitative Exercisewalking Programs* (New York: McGraw-Hill, 1990); Robert E. Thayer, *The Origin of Everyday Moods: Managing Energy, Tension, and Stress* (New York: Oxford University Press, 1996).

4. Deepak Chopra, *Perfect Health* (New York: Harmony Books, 1991), 262.

5. Joan Borysenko, with Larry Rothstein, *Minding the Body, Mending the Mind* (New York: Bantam Books, 1988), 9.

6. Thomas Moore, *The Re-Enchantment of Everyday Life* (New York: HarperCollins, 1996), ix.

7. Herbert Benson, with William Proctor, *Beyond the Relaxation Response* (New York: Times Books, 1984), 138.

## CHAPTER 2

1. Art Carey, "A Seasoned Strider Lives Up to Her Name," *Philadelphia Inquirer,* June 24, 1996, F1; Mary Walker, telephone conversations by the author, November 20, 1996, and October 27, 1997.

2. "Surgeon General's Report on Physical Activity and Health," *Journal of the American Medical Association* 276, no. 7 (Aug. 21, 1996): 522, reporting on "Physical Activity and Health: A Report of the Surgeon General," released July 11, 1996, by the Public

Health Service, U.S. Department of Health and Human Services.

3. Thayer, *The Origin of Everyday Moods,* 162.

4. Kathy Smith, with Susanna Levin, *Kathy Smith's WALKFIT for a Better Body* (New York: Warner Books, 1994), 16.

5. Thayer, *The Origin of Everyday Moods,* 191.

6. Target Heart Rate Chart adapted from: Kathleen Moloney and the Staff of the Canyon Ranch, *The Canyon Ranch Health and Fitness Program* (New York: Simon & Schuster, 1989), 78; Joyce D. Nash, Ph.D., *Maximize Your Body Potential* (Palo Alto, CA: Bull Publishing Company, 1986), 82; Robert Sweetgall, *Walk the Four Seasons* (Clayton, MO: Creative Walking, Inc., 1992), week 19; James M. Rippe, M.D., and Ann Ward, Ph.D., with Karla Dougherty, *The Rockport Walking Program* (New York: Prentice Hall Press, 1989).

7. Moloney and the Staff of the Canyon Ranch, *The Canyon Ranch Health and Fitness Program* (New York: Simon & Schuster, 1989), 78.

8. Shane Murphy, *The Achievement Zone* (New York: Putnam, 1996), 209–10. Based on work of G.A.V. Borg, "Perceived Exertion: A Note on History and Methods," *Medicine and Science in Sports and Exercise* 5 (1973), 90–93.

9. Bob Greene and Oprah Winfrey, *Make the Connection* (New York: Hyperion, 1996), 25.

10. Murphy, *The Achievement Zone,* 42. Telephone interview by the author, November 18, 1996.

11. Hal Borland, "To Own the Streets and Fields," *New York Times Magazine,* October 6, 1946. Reprinted by Aaron Sussman and Ruth Goode, *The Magic of Walking* (New York: Simon and Schuster, 1967), 312.

12. Dan Millman, *The Warrior Athlete: Body, Mind, and Spirit* (Walpole, NH: Stillpoint Publishing, 1979), 79.

13. Werner W. K. Hoeger, *Lifetime Physical Fitness and Wellness* (Englewood, CO: Morton, 1986), 127.

14. Chungliang Al Huang and Jerry Lynch, *Thinking Body, Dancing Mind: TaoSports for Extraordinary Performance in Athletics, Business, and Life* (New York: Bantam Books, 1992), 59.

## CHAPTER 3

1. Joe Henderson, "Foreword," in Kay Porter and Judy Foster, *The Mental Athlete* (Dubuque, IA: W. C. Brown, 1986), xi.
2. Linus Mundy, *Prayer-Walking* (St. Meinrad, IN: Abbey Press, 1994), ix.
3. Elton Richardson, telephone interview by author, May 21, 1996.
4. Benson, with Klipper, *The Relaxation Response*.
5. Benson, with Proctor, *Beyond the Relaxation Response*, 146.
6. Benson, with Stark, *Timeless Healing*, 135.
7. Shakti Gawain, *Creative Visualization* (New York: Bantam Books, 1982), 22.
8. Steven Levy, "Strip Mining the Corporate Life," *Newsweek* 128, no. 7 (Aug. 12, 1996): 54–55.
9. Al Huang and Lynch, *Thinking Body, Dancing Mind*, 31. Also, Douglas Bloch, *Words That Heal* (New York: Bantam Books, 1990), 83.

## CHAPTER 4

1. Steven Ungerleider, *Mental Training for Peak Performance* (Emmaus, PA: Rodale Press, 1996), 30–32. Telephone interview by author, December 10, 1996.
2. "Big Women Skip Exercise out of Fear of Ridicule," *The Register-Guard* (Eugene, OR), Dec. 18, 1996, 5D. Reporting on Pat Lyons, *Great Shape: The First Fitness Guide for Large Women* (Oakland, CA: Kaiser Permanente).
3. Porter and Foster, *The Mental Athlete*. Porter interviewed by author, Eugene, OR, December 6, 1996.

4. Shunryu Suzuki, *Zen Mind, Beginner's Mind* (New York: Weatherhill, 1970), 27.

5. Eknath Easwaran, *Meditation: An Eight-Point Program* (Petaluma, CA: Nilgiri Press, 1978), 57.

CHAPTER 5

1. Ungerleider, *Mental Training for Peak Performance,* 22.

2. James Joyce, "A Painful Case," *Dubliners* (New York: Viking, Compass Books Edition, 1958), 108.

3. Borysenko, with Rothstein, *Minding the Body, Mending the Mind,* 50.

4. Robert K. Cooper, *Health and Fitness Excellence* (Boston: Houghton Mifflin, 1989), 113.

5. Gawain, *Creative Visualization,* 6.

6. Suzuki, *Zen Mind, Beginner's Mind,* 25.

7. Stephanie Harris, board-certified neurologist, certified aerobics instructor, and continuing education provider for the American Council on Exercise and for Aerobics and Fitness Association of America. Interview by author, Eugene, OR, September 17, 1996.

8. Stephen Kiesling and E. C. Frederick, *Walk On: A Tool Kit for Building Your Own Walking Fitness Program* (Emmaus, PA: Rodale Press, 1986), 70.

9. Joseph Goldstein and Jack Kornfield, *Seeking the Heart of Wisdom: The Path of Insight Meditation* (Boston: Shambhala Dragon Editions, 1987), 195.

10. Tom Robbins, *Jitterbug Perfume* (New York: Bantam Books, 1984), 257.

CHAPTER 6

1. Benson, with Proctor, *Beyond the Relaxation Response,* 138.

2. Chopra, *The Seven Spiritual Laws of Success* (San Rafael, CA: Amber-Allen Publishing and New World Library, 1994), 13.

3. "Surgeon General's Report on Physical Activity and Health," 522.

4. Charles Porter, telephone interview by author, March 15, 1997.

5. Peace Pilgrim, *Peace Pilgrim: Her Life and Work in Her Own Words* (Santa Fe, NM: Ocean Tree Books, 1982), 26.

6. Pilgrim, *Peace Pilgrim,* 91.

7. Maggie Spilner, "A Beginner's Guide to Walking," *Prevention* 43, no. 3 (March 1993): 86.

8. Mari Messer, telephone interview by author, March 19, 1997.

9. Susan Freisinger, interview by author, Eugene, OR, August 19, 1996.

10. Lawrence LeShan, *How to Meditate* (Boston: Little, Brown, 1974), 55.

11. Jack Kornfield, *A Path with Heart* (New York: Bantam Books, 1993), 161.

12. Easwaran, *Meditation,* 29.

13. Terry Tempest Williams, *Pieces of White Shell: A Journey to Navajoland* (Albuquerque: University of New Mexico Press, 1984), 7.

14. Terence Monmaney, "Best Exercise Machine? It's the Simple Treadmill," *Los Angeles Times,* reprinted in *The Register-Guard,* May 6, 1996, A1. Reporting on a study published in the *Journal of the American Medical Association,* May 1996.

## CHAPTER 7

1. Al Huang and Lynch, *Thinking Body, Dancing Mind,* 89; Alan Watts, *The Wisdom of Insecurity* (New York: Pantheon Books, 1951), 130.

2. John J. L. Mood, *Rilke—On Love and Other Difficulties: Translations and Considerations of Rainer Maria Rilke* (New York: Norton, 1975), 99.

3. George Sheehan, "George Sheehan's Viewpoint," *Runner's World* 27, no. 8 (Aug. 1992), 20. Reprinted in Sheehan, *Going the Distance: One Man's Journey to the End of His Life* (New York: Villard, 1996), 66.

4. Benson, with Stark, *Timeless Healing,* 137.

5. Robert Frost, "A Servant to Servants," *The Poetry of Robert Frost* (New York: Holt, Rinehart and Winston, 1969), 64.

6. Harris, interview.

7. Benson, with Stark, *Timeless Healing,* 137.

8. Cheryl Brozovic, telephone interview by author, March 23, 1997.

9. Ann E. Boehler, "Walking Shorts: Musical Motivation," *Walking* 12, no. 2 (March–April 1997), 20.

10. Mark Fenton, "And the Beat Goes On . . . ", *Walking* 10, no. 1 (Jan.–Feb. 1995), 36.

11. Barbara De Angelis, *Real Moments* (New York: Delacorte Press, 1994), 238.

12. Gary Yanker and Kathy Burton, *Walking Medicine* (New York: McGraw-Hill, 1990), 219.

13. Dean Ornish, M.D., *Dr. Dean Ornish's Program for Reversing Heart Disease* (New York: Ballantine Books, 1990), 327.

14. Yanker and Burton, *Walking Medicine,* 219.

15. Kiesling and Frederick, *Walk On,* 30.

## CHAPTER 8

1. Stephanie Deer, interview by author, May 30, 1997.

2. Mark Bricklin, "With the Editor," *Prevention* 28, no. 5 (May 1996), 25. Cites research by James A. Blumenthal, Duke University.

3. Thayer, *The Origin of Everyday Moods,* 129, 187, 227.

4. Madeline Hersh, telephone interview by author, June 19, 1997.

5. *World Book Encyclopedia,* s. v. "Hippocrates." Mark Bricklin and Maggie Spilner, *Prevention's Practical Encyclopedia of Walking for Health* (Emmaus, PA: Rodale Press, 1992), 49.

6. Benson, with Stark, *Timeless Healing,* 272.

7. Sharon Stocker, with Denise Danford, "Well Versed," *Prevention* 48, no. 7 (July 1996), 93.

8. Mundy, *Prayer-Walking,* 51.

9. Eugene Guillevic, "The Task," *Selected Poems,* trans. by Denise Levertov (New York: New Directions, 1969), 137.

10. Sam Gill, "Navajo Nightway Prayer," *Native American Traditions* (Belmont, CA: Wadsworth, 1983), 56.

11. May Sarton, "The Invocation to Kali," *A Grain of Mustard Seed (1967–1971)* (New York: Norton, 1971), 23.

12. Cited in M. J. Ryan, ed., *A Grateful Heart* (Berkeley, CA: Conari Press, 1994), 171.

13. Elizabeth Roberts and Elias Amidon, eds., "Inuit Song," *Earth Prayers from Around the World* (San Francisco: HarperSanFrancisco, 1991), 41.

14. Kay Gilley, *Leading from the Heart* (Boston: Butterworth-Heinemann, 1996), 106–7. Telephone interview by author, March 19, 1997.

15. Carolyn Scott Kortge, "Taken to the Cleaners," "My Turn," *Newsweek* 126, no. 17 (Oct. 23, 1995), 16.

## CHAPTER 9

1. René Daumal, "Postface," *Mount Analogue,* trans. by Roger Shattuck (San Francisco, CA: City Lights Books, 1959), 103.

2. Margo Chisholm, telephone interview by author, May 16, 1997.

3. Margo Chisholm and Ray Bruce, *To the Summit* (New York: Avon, 1997), 59.

4. Chisholm and Bruce, *To the Summit,* 61.

5. Colin Fletcher, *The Secret Worlds of Colin Fletcher* (New York: Knopf, 1989), 7.

6. Mark Black, interview by author, Tucson, AZ, June 10, 1996.

7. Thich Nhat Hanh, "A Guide to Walking Meditation," from a videotape filmed at Green Gulch Zen Center, CA. (Berkeley, CA: Parallax Press), available from Sounds True, Boulder, CO.

8. Thich Nhat Hanh, *The Long Road Turns to Joy: A Guide to Walking Meditation,* 15.

9. Marsha Sinetar, *A Way Without Words* (Mahwah, NJ: Paulist Press, 1992), 21.

10. James Swan, telephone interview by author, May 27, 1997.

11. Henri Frédéric Amiel, "What a Lovely Walk," *The Private Journal of Henri Frédéric Amiel,* trans. by Van Wyck Brooks and Charles Van Wyck Brooks, reprinted in Aaron Sussman and Ruth Goode, *The Magic of Walking,* (New York: Simon and Schuster, 1967), 300.

12. Thich Nhat Hanh, "The Path Is You," *The Long Road Turns to Joy: A Guide to Walking Meditation* (Berkeley, CA: Parallax Press, 1996), 72.

13. Rainer Maria Rilke, "Eingang" ("The Way In"), *Selected Poems of Rainer Maria Rilke,* trans. by Robert Bly (New York: Harper & Row, 1981), 71.

## CHAPTER 10

1. Norman Nicholson, ed., *The Lake District: An Anthology* (Harmondsworth, England: Penguin Books, 1978), 25. Reprinted from Daniel Dafoe, *A Tour Through the Whole Island of Great Britain,* published in three volumes, 1724–27.

2. Bill Bryson, "Beauty Besieged: England's Lake District," *National Geographic* 189, no. 2 (Aug. 1994), 11.

3. Peter Matthiessen, *The Snow Leopard* (New York: Bantam Books, 1979), 238.

4. Matthiessen, *The Snow Leopard,* 239.

5. Pilgrim, *Peace Pilgrim,* 27.

6. Pilgrim, *Peace Pilgrim,* 25.

7. Pilgrim, *Peace Pilgrim,* 33.

8. Gordon Klatt, telephone interview by author, July 7, 1997.

9. Alison Raju, *The Way of Saint James: Spain* (Milnthorpe, Cumbria, Great Britain: Cicerone Press, 1994), 9.

10. Keith Sugden, *Walking the Pilgrim Ways* (Newton Abbot, Devon, Great Britain: David & Charles, 1991), 6.

11. Raju, *The Way of Saint James: Spain,* 13, 17.

12. Millán Bravo Lozano, "The Road to Compostela," *The UNESCO Courier,* 48, (May 1995), 21–23.

13. Sugden, *Walking the Pilgrim Ways,* 102–17.

14. Christopher Portway, *Journey Along the Spine of the Andes* (Sparkford, Yeovil, Somerset, England: Oxford Illustrated Press, 1984), 11–19.

15. Appalachian Mountain Club, *AMC White Mountain Guide, 25th Edition* (Boston: Appalachian Mountain Club, 1992), xxxi.

16. James Carse, telephone interview by author, July 14, 1997.

17. "The Talk of the Town," *The New Yorker,* 69, no. 33, (Oct. 11, 1993), 43.

18. Ralph Waldo Emerson, "Nature," *The Best of Ralph Waldo Emerson* (Roslyn, NY: Walter J. Black, 1941), 108.

19. Emerson, "Nature," 100.

20. Swan, telephone interview by author.

21. Thomas Merton, *The Silent Life* (New York: Farrar, Straus & Giroux, 1957), 167.

# ACKNOWLEDGMENTS

Enormous gratitude permeates this book. It was created in a spirit of joyful appreciation for recovery of a sense of wholeness, for discovery of meditation in movement, and for spiritual connection in nature. It attests to the support and encouragement of many people who have accompanied my steps along the route that led to this place of thanksgiving:

To the enthusiastic walkers and researchers who agreed to share their own discoveries and experiences in interviews, I give thanks for trust in my vision and for bringing wisdom and breadth to this book.

To the mentors, editors, colleagues, sources, and readers who helped mold my sense of journalistic integrity, I give thanks for professional skills and for courage and compassion.

To the coaches, training partners, and competitors who taught me the joy of athletic expression, I give thanks for a disciplined practice that treats the body as partner, rather than container.

To the Carmelite nuns at the Carmel of Maria Regina, I give thanks for spiritual sisterhood and for introducing me to the concept of constant prayer.

To the Buddhist nuns in the Kagyu Droden Kunchab three-year retreat, I give thanks for greeting this project with a resounding benediction: "May all beings benefit."

To Natalie Goldberg, author of *Writing Down the Bones,* I give thanks for expanding my definition of spiritual practice.

To Catherine Harris, bookseller and spiritual trailblazer, I give thanks for launching me into this book with admonitions to write, not talk.

To Elizabeth Lyon, freelance editor and author of *Nonfiction Book Proposals Anybody Can Write,* I give thanks for assistance in developing a proposal that got the attention of Tom Grady at HarperSanFrancisco. For unwavering demands for clarity, I give thanks to members of the Tuesday Writers' Group: Geraldine Moreno-Black, DeLora Jenkins, Cynthia Pappas, Elsie Rochna, Mabel Armstrong, Maura Conlon-McIvor, Ann Fuller, Kiernan Phipps, Candy Davis.

To Caroline Pincus and Sally Kim at HarperSanFrancisco, I give thanks for reassurance, stability, and professional excellence. To Nancy Palmer Jones, I offer gratitude for an extraordinarily caring copyedit of the manuscript.

To Vicky Ayers I give thanks for quiet companionship on walks and for the calm, unwavering support that cradled the conception of this book and helped me stay on course.

To Christy Tinker, Mary Ellen Bishop, and José McCarthy, I give thanks for weekly assistance in transforming aspirations into action.

To Rosanne Olson and Ted McMahan, and to Barbara and John Mundall, I give thanks for enduring friendship, tolerance, and encouragement through two years of single-minded obsession. Rosanne's photographic artistry and Ted's poetic sensitivity as first reader of the manuscript made an enormous contribution.

To my husband, Dean Kortge, I give thanks for the generosity of spirit and for the sustaining love, support, and companionship that have freed me to travel a creative path and to reach this joyful junction of walking and writing. I am forever and deeply grateful that you choose to walk beside me.

# INDEX

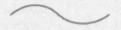

Page numbers in *italics* refer to illustrations.